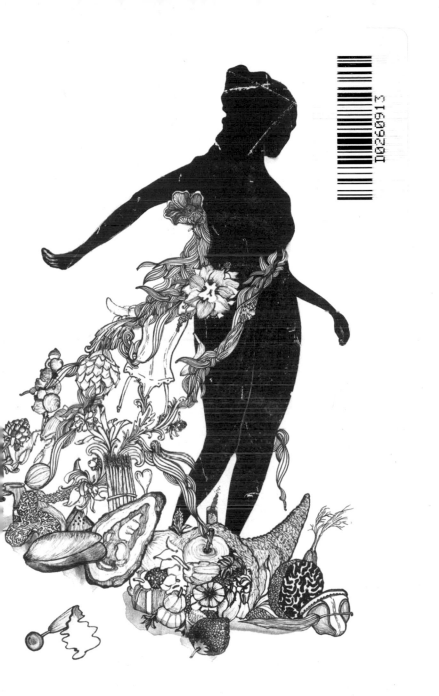

D0260913

THE
APHRODISIAC
ENCYCLOPAEDIA

THE
APHRODISIAC
ENCYCLOPAEDIA

*A Gourmet Guide
to Culinary Come-Ons*

MARK DOUGLAS HILL

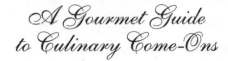

SQUARE PEG

Published by Square Peg 2011

10 9 8 7 6 5 4 3 2 1

Copyright © Mark Douglas Hill 2011

The Author has asserted his rights under the Copyright, Designs
and Patents Act 1988 to be identified as the author of this work

This book is sold subject to the condition that it shall not,
by way of trade or otherwise, be lent, resold, hired out, or otherwise
circulated without the publisher's prior consent in any form of
binding or cover other than that in which it is published and without
a similar condition, including this condition, being imposed
on the subsequent purchaser

First published in Great Britain in 2011 by
Square Peg
Random House, 20 Vauxhall Bridge Road,
London SW1V 2SA

www.rbooks.co.uk

Addresses for companies within The Random House Group Limited can be found at:
www.randomhouse.co.uk/offices.htm

The Random House Group Limited Reg. No. 954009

A CIP catalogue record for this book
is available from the British Library

ISBN 978 0 224 08697 4

The Random House Group Limited supports The Forest Stewardship Council (FSC),
the leading international forest certification organisation. All our titles that are
printed on Greenpeace approved FSC certified paper carry the FSC logo. Our paper
procurement policy can be found at www.randomhouse.co.uk/environment

Mixed Sources
Product group from well-managed
forests and other controlled sources
www.fsc.org Cert no. TT-COC-2139
© 1996 Forest Stewardship Council
FSC

Designed by Nicky Barneby @ Barneby Ltd
Printed and bound in Great Britain by MPG Books Ltd, Bodmin, Cornwall

To long lunches and lie-ins – and everyone who enjoys them.

Acknowledgements

The Aphrodisiac Encyclopaedia would simply not have been possible without the hard work and help of many people. They are too many to mention but particular thanks go to Jenny McVeigh who got the ball rolling, Tim Glister at Janklow and my wonderful editor at Square Peg, Rosemary Davidson. The support, advice and patience of friends and family has also been invaluable. Lots of love to Fred and Jessica, Claire, Jane and Julian and, above all, Atalanta.

Contents

Introduction

The pleasures of the table and delights of the boudoir are my *raison d'être*. Without these very pillars of existence my lot would be grim and grey indeed. For I am a bon viveur: an epicurean, glutton, sybarite and sensualist – and damn proud of it too!

I have spent a lifetime diligently in pursuit of all the good things life has to offer. The world has been my oyster and I have slurped it down and bellowed for more. To my dismay, I observe that an exuberant enjoyment of gastronomy does not always prelude a postprandial degustation of more fleshly delights. In fact, all too frequently, and terribly regrettably, a heavy meal is a wet blanket on the fire of desire. Thankfully, it does not have to be this way. One can have one's cake and eat it. Far from extinguishing passion, there are some blessed ingredients that actively incite a digestive tumbling: foods that encourage friskiness and enhance the frisking. I am referring to what are commonly known as aphrodisiacs.

Aphrodisiacs intrigue me. Over the years I have researched and refined, trialled and tested ingredients and recipes from all over the world. I have experienced smells, tastes and sensations from near and far, the memories of which rise unbidden at unguarded moments. Flowery Turkish delight over a solitary narghile in the Grand Bazaar of Istanbul; fresh sea urchin aboard my yacht, bobbing on the Adriatic; roast iguana in the Yucatán served up by a Mayan mama in a jungle hut; an oozing mango plucked in the primordial rainforest of the remote Andaman Islands. A midnight feast of vintage champagne and royal beluga caviar prepared by an alabaster princess in St Petersburg; mouth-tingling puffer-fish sashimi shared with some shady Yakuza in a dark Tokyo nightclub. From high society to the demi-monde, from the exquisitely refined to the frankly savage, I have tucked in regardless. The pursuit of pleasure is a passport to strange places and stranger faces. It has taken me on a merry dance. I have dined and dallied to my heart's content, sowing wild oats with enthusiastic abandon. Modesty forbids too much candour; suffice to say my efforts have never been met with anything short of ecstatic approval and total satisfaction. Now in my twilight years I have dedicated myself to the catalogue of my experiences, and the creation of this compendium. A veritable smorgasbord of aphrodisiacs, it will be a gift to future generations, the legacy of a lifetime's research, a reference and resource to aid, abet and amuse the bon viveurs of tomorrow.

Aphrodisiacs have been a preoccupation of man since the dawn of time. Civilisations, from ancient to modern, have sought to enhance their sexual experience, experimenting with substances ranging from the everyday and delicious to the truly bizarre and positively disgusting. The list includes such unappetising eccentricities as whale's bile, embryonic eggs and pulverised beetles. In my encyclopaedia I have ignored these culinary abominations, focusing my efforts exclusively on those truly edible aphrodisiacs. Ingredients one can consume with genuine gastronomic pleasure. Also off the menu are the body parts of rare animals. There is a time and a place for a tiger's penis. That place is a frisky lady tiger under a full moon. It is not in a steaming bowl of oriental soup.

Edible, ethical or otherwise, aphrodisiacs enjoy mythic reputations. These magical properties, however, remain shrouded in mystery and distinctly metaphysical. My aim is to untangle truth from tittle-tattle and lift this fog of confusion. The application of science and nutritional know-how has sifted pretender from contender, identifying and illuminating the empirical evidence underpinning aphrodisiac reputations. The final flourish is a soupçon of culinary creativity unleashed in a set of stylish yet simple recipes. A user's guide to unlock the amorous and gastronomic potential of each featured aphrodisiac. No pot has been left unstirred, no titbit untried or delicacy undevoured.

I welcome you to these pages. Dig in and delight in the dainties unearthed. Diversion, deviation and delectation await.

Bon appétit!

Author's Note
All recipes serve two

Alcohol

I T SEEMS INCREASINGLY true that without the miracle of alcohol there would be no sex. Mankind would surely founder in a bog of inconsequential small talk and missed sexual opportunity. In our increasingly sedate and sterile world, a skinful of booze has become the ultimate aphrodisiac. Euripides, the great Greek tragedian, hit the nail on the head in 405 BC, professing with the righteous passion of a tipsy playwright that 'if wine ceases, there will be an end of Love, an end to every pleasure in the life of man'. And the man has a point, for cast your mind over your own sexual escapades and count yourself unusual indeed if you can honestly say that alcohol played no part in proceedings.

Producing alcohol is one of man's oldest and most enduring preoccupations. The ancient Egyptians were early pioneers, developing detailed hieroglyphic recipes for the production of beer and wine. Enjoyed at all social occasions, booze lubricated both social and spiritual life. The Greeks expanded this tradition of tippling with the cult of Dionysus (also known as Bacchus), god of wine and wildness. After dark, deep in the wilderness, celebrants would gather to commune with their god, freeing themselves from the constraints of civilisation with wine, wild drumming, frenzied dancing and ecstatic copulation. Distillation originated in India; gradually percolating westwards it gave rise to brandy and whisky in the early Middle Ages. From this time on the variety of alcohol available to the amorous of intention has ballooned to a bewildering array of beers, wines, spirits and liqueurs, each with its own specific quirks and qualities.

Despite its bawdy reputation, the physiological and psychological reality is that alcohol can turn from a potent aphrodisiac into the exact opposite. The key, rather boringly, is moderation. Alcohol's wildly divergent effect directly depends on the degree of one's drunkenness, just as likely to result in a snoring stupor as a bed-breaking bout of bonking. Mild inebriation is most typified by a euphoric state characterised by increased confidence, sociability and good humour. Under the influence, inhibitions are shrugged off. Self-restraint weakens whilst coordination remains more or less intact: so far, so good. Imbibe further and things start to unravel surprisingly swiftly. The carouser enters a state of excitement, experiencing emotional instability, loss of critical judgement and impairment of perception, memory and cognition. Poor judgement, blurred vision and an equally annihilated adversary might just lead to an enthusiastic fumble on the dance floor. Try for a quick round of hide-the-sausage, however, and one will sadly find one's supposed saveloy distinctly chipolata. Needless to say, drinking more will assist neither seduction nor sexual congress and should remain firmly the preserve of drowning sorrows.

Science strongly supports moderation. Obtuse as ever, most of us cling to the conviction that excess alcohol is the key to carnal delights. In a way we are right. Several bottles of plonk may not score the proverbial home run but they could be the necessary crutch in a hobble to first base. The sober mind cowers at the crushing consequence of possible rejection. Advances are almost unthinkable without a large measure of Dutch courage. Equally strongly engrained is the belief that almost certain rejection can be evaded only by pickling the object of our affection. Indeed, the enthusiasm with which a date submits to said sousing is often a suitor's best guide to amorous availability; five shots of tequila sends signals that a small white wine spritzer somehow does not.

COCKTAILS

To my mind the best way to win hearts and minds through alcohol is via the medium of cocktails. You can tailor a cocktail to your companion's tastes, suavely prepare it with an arsenal of shiny chrome gadgets, name it after them and still sneak a gallon of hard liquor into a drink that mysteriously tastes no stronger than lemonade. One such suave seducer is the Rose Petal Martini, heady with the floral bouquet of horticulture's most sensual bloom. Serve in iced Martini glasses sprinkled with rose petals, easy on the eye and even easier on the tongue. Ladies should look no further than a Dirty Vodka Martini, mastery of which should be all that is needed to unleash a man's licence to thrill.

....

Dirty Vodka Martini
Ice : Plenty
Vodka (Belvedere) : 100ml
Olive brine : 1 tbsp
Dry vermouth (Noilly Prat) : 1 tbsp
Green queen olive (brined) : 1

As this drink is essentially pure vodka, the quality of the vodka is paramount. My Martini vodka of choice is Belvedere, which is smoother than Roger Moore himself. To prepare the cocktail, first place your Martini glass in the freezer. Fill a cocktail shaker with ice and pour over it four 25ml shots of vodka, a tablespoonful of olive brine and ½ a shot of dry white vermouth, and my preference is for Noilly Prat. Although Mr Bond is firmly pro shake, I am a staunch stirrer when it comes to Martinis, which unlike shaking guarantees a clear cocktail. Thirty seconds to a minute of stirring should suffice. Strain the mixed cocktail into your iced Martini glass, garnish with a large green queen olive, and serve with a smouldering look.

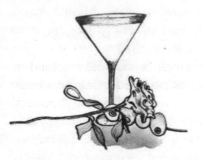

Rose Petal Martini

Ice : Plenty
Vodka (Belvedere) : 3 shots
Rose syrup : 1 shot
Angostura bitters : 1 dash
Dry vermouth : ½ shot
Fresh rose petals : 2
Lemon peel : 8 cm length

*Following the same drill as for the vodka Martini, chill your
Martini glasses and fill a cocktail shaker with ice. Pour over 3
measures of Belvedere vodka, 1 measure of rose syrup, a dash
of Angostura bitters and ½ a measure of dry vermouth.
Stir for a minute, then strain into your chilled glasses and
garnish with a couple of perfect rose petals and a twist of lemon
peel. If you cannot lay your hands on rose syrup (look out for
Monin's), you can use Lanique's rose liqueur or simply make your
own by steeping ½ a cup of dried rose petals in a cup of water
with a cup of sugar. Leave overnight and strain out the petals.*

CHAMPAGNE

Be it a white wedding in the Shires or a sordid weekend in
Pigalle, no beverage offers quite the same romantic possibility
as a chilled bottle of bubbly. Champagne roars of sauciness,
seduction and sex. Its exorbitant price, the weighty foiled
and fettered bottle, the rituals, paraphernalia and efferves-
cent intoxication — everything about champagne is deeply
suggestive.

The seeds for champagne's lofty reputation were sown in the
Dark Ages. In 496 AD the barbarian king Clovis I was baptised in
Reims, capital of the champagne region. The affair was rather
miraculous, involving a dove sent from heaven, a sacred phial
of oil and a saintly bishop. It also proved to have momentous
consequences as Clovis went on to unite France under Catholi-
cism and become its first king. Reims has been the ceremonial
location for the coronation of French kings ever since. At the

coronation after-parties the tipple *du jour* has always been the local brew – champagne.

The wine enjoyed by Clovis and his cronies would have little in common with that of today. The first innovation, widely attributed to Dom Pérignon, was the creation of bubbles. Cellar master at the monastery of Épernay in the late seventeenth century, he started bottling the local wine before fermentation was complete. The gas released by the ongoing fermentation was reabsorbed, creating champagne's now trademark fizz. This development was perfected in the nineteenth century with the secondary fermentation of the *méthode champenoise*. The final innovation was the emergence of the dry style of modern champagne. This dates back to 1846 when Perrier-Jouët decided not (or perhaps forgot) to sweeten the wine bound for England. The English loved it and in 1872 the brut style of champagne was officially recognised and modern champagne was born. Cheers and bottoms up to that.

It is easy to attribute champagne's aphrodisiac allure to its social status: a universal shorthand for success, luxury and celebration. This no doubt plays a placebo part in proceedings but isn't to my mind the whole story. The rituals involved in champagne are undeniably sultry. There is a pent-up energy and tension in the heavy reinforced bottle, a teasing provocation in the undressing and unwiring of the bottle's phallic neck and bulbous cork. The release is metaphoric, either sudden with a foamy jet of excitement, or controlled as the pressure is released with the whimper of the '*soupir amoureux*'. Once in a glass and in one's mouth, the yeasty fragrance, tingle of bubbles and cool acidity are both invigorating and intoxicating. And really it is intoxicating, a hefty 12–13 per cent of alcohol which those delightful bubbles mainline straight to the brain.

Socially and psychologically, champagne's aphrodisiac reputation glitters convincingly. There is also a bit of science behind the sparkle. Champagne packs a poky punch of aphrodisiac trace minerals. These include potassium, zinc and magnesium, all absolutely essential for both male and female sex hormone production. It is also said that the yeasty bouquet of dry champagne accurately mimics the scent of female sex pheromones. Probably why rock stars are compelled to fill bathtubs and bathe in the stuff.

Selecting champagne is a rather delicate process. The various brands are closely associated with quite disparate social tribes. The hip-hop fraternity has a decided penchant for Cristal. The posh prefer the well-bred orange of Veuve Clicquot, whilst the nouveau get off on Moët or Laurent-Perrier. Winston Churchill drank Pol Roger and the Queen tipples on Taittinger. The bon viveur, however, sides with the bone-dry, rich and well-mannered Bollinger – just like James Bond. Chill Bolly to around 8 degrees (not too frosty), and if you are peckish pass on the strawberries and serve with a side portion of caviar, scrambled eggs and potato latkes.

It would be sacrilege to adulterate a top-drawer vintage champagne with anything other than one's tongue. At the entry level of the market, however, there is much to be said for fortifying and fancifying less exalted champagnes into extravagant cocktails. Almost everything has been mixed with champagne from stout in Black Velvet to blackcurrant liqueur in Kir Royale.

My preference is to keep the cocktail clean and classic whilst adding a little extra alcoholic va-va-voom and seductive spice. The Vanilla Thriller ticks the boxes. Like all good cocktails it is fun and frivolous yet decidedly feisty.

. . . .

Vanilla Thriller Champagne Cocktail

Vanilla : ¼ pod
Brandy : 1 shot
Sugar cube : 1
Angostura bitters : 2 shakes
Dry non-vintage champagne : 1 bottle

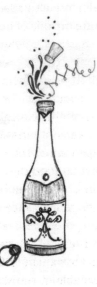

Simple enough for the prettiest to prepare: split the vanilla pod, scrape out the seeds and mix them with the brandy. Place the sugar cube in the bottom of a champagne glass and saturate with the Angostura bitters. Add the vanilla brandy and top up with champagne. As you sip away at the cocktail, the layers will mix, giving a stronger vanilla flavour as you descend the glass.

. . . .

RED WINE

Very occasionally a bon viveur must rein in that urge to splurge – if only to refresh the appetite for new indulgence. When the abstemious mood strikes, exile from alcohol seems to reliably satisfy the inner ascetic. Red wine is of course allowed, for as every right-thinking person knows, red wine is medicinal. Comprehensively hailed as good for the heart, red wine now appears quite capable of quickening the pulse too.

A study of 789 women in Florence found rather conclusively that, for these women at least, red wine and libido were amorously entwined. One group drank a couple of glasses of red wine a day, a second group drank less than a glass a day of any alcoholic drink, a third group was teetotal. All the women answered a series of indelicate questions assessing how often they wanted sexy time, how easily they became aroused and how satisfied they were with their sexual experiences. The red winos swept the board, significantly lustier than the satisfactory performance of the regular boozers; the teetotal crawled home a distant and somewhat frustrated last.

The active ingredient giving red wine its carnal edge is an antioxidant called resveratrol. Uniquely and abundantly available in the skin of red grapes, resveratrol is able to stop the natural conversion of the libido-driving male sex hormone testosterone into the less voracious feminine hormone oestrogen. Both sexes produce both hormones; however, in women testosterone levels are much lower and sexual appetite more finely tuned to its fluctuation. In men, red wine and resveratrol have the clearest effect during the mysterious male menopause. Testosterone levels drop and the conversion into oestrogen speeds up. The most visible symptom of the male menopause is the sudden development of the middle-aged male mammary or 'moob'. Fight the 'moob' and maintain manly mojo with red wine regularly.

Having science on your side is always nice but red wine's appeal runs deeper. A glass of good claret spreads a warm glow throughout the body. The nuances of flavour and rich bouquet awaken the senses and suffuse sensuality. When it comes to selecting a seductive red, it is old world and old money all the way. Nothing fits the bill better than the pure Merlot, Right Bank clarets of Pomerol. Fortifying wine with spices has long been held as a way to enhance wine's aphrodisiac effect. French author Rabelais champions a Burgundy-based brew in *Gargantua and Pantagruel*. *Hippocras Aphrodisiac* is spiced and sweetened with ginger, cinnamon, cloves, vanilla and sugar. *Aqua Mirabilis*, a splendidly named and similarly fortified wine, was a favourite of Louis XIV. This version mixes cinnamon, galangal, ginger, nutmeg, rosemary and thyme with claret. The concoction is left to mature for a week and then strained. When it comes to spiced wine my mind naturally turns to mulled wine. My version is unusual in that it uses a ruby port base, which itself has a particularly aphrodisiac reputation.

Mulled Port Mirabilis

Grated nutmeg : ½
Fresh ginger : 4 cm length
Ruby port : 1 bottle
Ground cinnamon : 1 tsp
Cloves : 1 tsp
Rosemary : 2 fresh sprigs
Thyme : 3 fresh sprigs
Honey : to taste

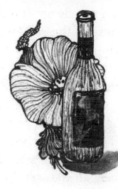

*The beauty of this recipe is that the mulled wine needs no
fortification, and less sweetening than a traditional mulled wine.
However, it does require a little advance preparation. First grate
the nutmeg and finely chop the fresh ginger. Sample a little of
the ruby port, then add all the spices and herbs to the bottle.
Shake vigorously and leave to infuse for one week. Strain the port
into a saucepan to remove all the spices and heat gently. Taste
for sweetness and if required add a teaspoon or so of honey.
Serve on a chilly night to warm cockles and muscles for an
amorous encounter.*

Fruit

BANANA

Whilst few healthy men's underpants house a bright yellow fellow, in other respects the banana is a dead ringer for the male appendage. The general proportions and gentle curve of the banana are so redolent of man's best friend that it would be surprising if bananas were not considered aphrodisiacs.

Cultivated for over six thousand years, as bananas have spread from South-East Asia across the globe so has their steamy reputation. In Central America locals knock back the sap of the red banana tree to fortify themselves for nights of passion. In India, the banana is considered a powerful fertility symbol which wannabe lotharios offer to the gods to aid their amorous endeavours. Although the jury is still out on the reliability of these two particular practices, there are plenty of reasons to suppose that eating a banana or two before engaging in some adult acrobatics is rather a good idea.

Bananas contain the amino acid tryptophan, which the body metabolises into serotonin, also known as the 'molecule of happiness'. The loved-up feeling ravers enjoy when they pop an E is the body dumping its reserves of serotonin into the bloodstream. Conversely, low serotonin levels are an almost symptomatic feature of depression. I have correspondingly noted that whilst loved-up ravers get frisky at the drop of a jester's hat, the depressed tend to go home alone. Bananas also ape the effects of another Class A narcotic naughty, cocaine. Eating bananas stimulates the release of dopamine, the body's impulse and reward pleasure hormone. We crave this stuff above all else, driving us to do whatever it takes to get our fix. Sex is hard-wired into our brains to give the biggest fix of all. Once we detect increased dopamine levels swilling around the brain, the waves of pleasure easily lead to sexual arousal. Indeed, medicinal drugs that increase dopamine levels (to counter ADHD for example) have the well-documented side effect of supercharging the sex drive.

It seems that bananas not only put one in a decidedly rude mood but can also improve performance should you want to take things horizontal. They contain the enzyme bromelain, which as well as being used to tenderise meat also has the possibly related but infinitely more useful property of lengthening a man's countdown to blast-off. Luckily the banana's triple whammy of natural sugars (sucrose, fructose and glucose) provides an instant and sustained source of energy to accompany one's improved restraint. Apparently two bananas pack enough punch to power a ninety-minute workout, though I am sure one banana would be enough for all but the most ardently in love. The final piece of the banana's nutritional jigsaw is a healthy wallop of vitamin B6, which boosts semen production and stimulates the production of sex hormones in both men and women, keeping libidos lively and people smiley.

Bananas are the most widely consumed fruit in the world, and the world widely consumes them in their natural state. When I think of bananas I am mainly thinking of breakfast; they kick-start the day with a hit of instant energy, and put you in a good mood to boot. Slice into a bowl of granola with a dollop of yoghurt and a splash of milk in the summer, or add to a bowl of steaming oatmeal in winter – hard to beat if it's a healthy breakfast you want. Alternatively, blend with low-fat yoghurt, a little apple juice, some dates, a spoonful of granola and a dollop of honey – a liquid breakfast that will last you all the way to lunch and won't give you indigestion should you engage in any vigorous activity shortly after consumption.

....

Glorious Morning Smoothie
Apple juice : 100 ml
Low fat yoghurt : 200 ml
Banana : 1
Chopped dates : 2 tbsp
Granola : 2 tbsp (see p 220)
Honey : to taste

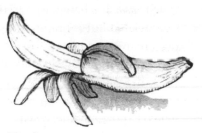

*It couldn't be easier thanks
to the wonders of modern
technology. Equip yourself with a blender,
put all the ingredients in the jug and press the button. Slurp
down the resulting goo, take off your pyjamas and take on
the world.*

....

DURIAN

The tropics of South-East Asia are an outlandish and intoxicating place for the travelling gourmet. Confronted with a stinking serving of fresh durian flesh, this will seem especially true. To the uninitiated this is the most unlikely of aphrodisiacs. Uncommon in the West, in Indonesia the durian is revered as the 'king of fruits'. It is voraciously consumed across South-East Asia. Durians are enormous and look distinctly forbidding. A formidable husk of green thorns covers an abstract oblong fruit, which can grow over 30 centimetres long and weigh a hefty 3 kilograms. It is only when you break open the husk to reveal the edible flesh that the durian's poky pong is fully deployed. Trumping an overripe Vacherin by some margin, the aroma of durian is strong, penetrating and, to many, absolutely abhorrent. Even in its Indonesian homeland, this king of fruits is something of a pariah, *non grata* on public transport and in most hotels.

The smell is beyond description, a fetid combination of almonds, rotten onions, turpentine and old trainer. Nothing about this smell encourages the novice to actually taste the fruit. The flavour that rewards the intrepid is something of a surprise, in that it is surprisingly pleasant. Five satin cells of firm creamy pulp form the edible part of the durian. They have a unique silky smooth texture with an equally unique almond-custard flavour with nuances of cream cheese, sherry and caramelised onion. Richard Burton, the Victorian sensualist and explorer, describes the fruit as 'neither acid nor sweet nor juicy, yet it wants neither of these qualities, for it is in itself perfect. It produces no nausea or other bad effect, and the more you eat of it the less you feel inclined to stop. In fact, to eat Durians is a new sensation worth a voyage to the East to experience.' Add to Burton's eulogy possible aphrodisiac effects and that trip East is increasingly enticing.

The Javanese are the most fervent advocates of the durian's amorous efficacy. For the average Javan gentleman the proverb '*durian jatuh sarung naik*' ('when the durians fall, the sarongs come up') is more fact than folklore. There is even a set of rules of what and what not to eat after durian to control its libidinous urges. Durian is an undeniably sensual eating experience. The fruit's silky texture is a sybarite's wet dream. The rich, intense flavour equals the complexity of a fine wine. There is something intangibly alluring about the fruit's impressive size and girth. However, the real origins of durian's rampant reputation lie deep in the primeval Indonesian rainforest. The beasts of the forest go dotty for durian. Elephants, orang-utans, monkeys, deer, pigs and even tigers will travel large distances to get some. It is believed that this beast-beloved fruit can connect its human devotees to an ancient animalistic instinct, invoking the spirit of Orang Pendek, the tropical Indonesian Bigfoot.

There is substantial nutritional evidence to support the durian effect. High in vitamin C, sugar and potassium, durian also has peculiarly high levels of oestrogens and the amino acid tryptophan. Tryptophan metabolises into serotonin which, as we saw with bananas, creates cresting waves of extreme pleasure when released into the brain following certain ecstatic moments; the more serotonin, the more tidal that wave of pleasure. When it comes to durians, Western science and Chinese medicine are in unusual accord. According to Chinese food classification, durian is one of a handful of raw foods that create 'heat'. As such it is seen as a yang or male force tonic, able to strengthen and replenish the qi vigour that governs libido and is lost in ejaculation. Not bad for a big stinky fruit banned from public transport.

Preparing an alluring dish of durian is something of a challenge. It is hard to tame its dubious fragrance. Perhaps rather obviously, durian is best served al fresco. Sit your dining companion upwind and serve your durian as a dessert. By this time senses will have been mellowed by previous courses, adventure aroused by a drink or two. The durian's gastronomic strength is its complex exotic flavour and sensual texture, so it makes sense to serve it simply in its unadulterated raw form. It is delicious to both devotee and debutante as part of a fruit salad of mango and raspberries. The mango complements the durian's texture whilst the tartness of the raspberries cuts through its creamy richness. Accompany with a dramatic black rice pudding, rich and sticky with coconut. Garnish with toasted coconut flakes and prepare for tropical paradise and jungle fever.

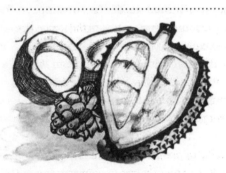

Durian Fruit Salad and Black Coconut Rice Pudding

Black sweet rice : 100 g
Mango : 1 ripe medium-sized fruit
Durian : 1 lobe
Chambord (raspberry liqueur) 1 tbsp
Raspberries : 150 g

Coconut milk : 100 ml
Brown sugar : 50 g / to taste
Salt : to taste
Toasted coconut flakes : 1 tsp

If you can't find sticky black rice use standard sticky white rice.
Place the rice in a non-stick saucepan and cover with water. Swill
it around to wash and dislodge any loose husks. Skim the loose
husks, then drain the rice and return to the dish.

Add 600 ml of water to the rice and bring to the boil over
a high heat. Reduce the heat and simmer until the rice is soft
(around 45 minutes), stirring occasionally. Meanwhile cut the
stone from the ripe mango and chop the flesh into 2 cm cubes.
Cut the durian flesh into similar-sized chunks. Pour over the
Chambord raspberry liqueur and gently mix with the washed
raspberries. Leave to macerate.

Once the rice is soft, drain off any excess water so that the
level is just below that of the cooked rice. Add the coconut
milk, sugar and a couple of good pinches of salt to the rice and
simmer, stirring frequently until the rice pudding reaches a thick
creamy consistency.

To serve, place a ladleful of rice pudding in the centre of a
warmed plate. Shake a little so that the rice pudding spreads out
to form a circle. Place a pile of fruit salad in the centre of the rice
pudding. Dress with a little of the macerating juice and garnish
with a sprinkling of toasted coconut flakes.

FIG

Figs are part of the aphrodisiac establishment. Breaking open an oozingly ripe fig and eating it out is quite rightly regarded as downright saucy, highly suggestive of an intimate oral act between a man and a woman. The fig's contours are strikingly testicular; its inverted flower anatomy positively womby. Such visual sexual stimulus did not escape early man's lascivious leer and the fig has been a symbol for fornication and fecundity almost for ever.

The ancient Greeks dedicated the fig to the lusty and heroically endowed god Dionysus, who was represented at licentious all-night revels by a giant phallus carved from fig wood. In Roman times the fig tree was sacred to Priapus, god of procreation and the wide-awake winky. Even today the medical term for an uncontrollable and pathologically sustained erection is 'priapism'. The fig was equally pervasive as a symbol for feminine fertility, appearing on monuments with the letter delta and a barleycorn as part of the *Concha Veneris*, or Delta of Venus. Given the fig's X-rated ancient pedigree and her mythic nymphomania, it is no surprise that they were also one of Cleopatra's favourite snacks.

The most offensive ancient Greek gesture was to make a fist and lewdly extend your middle finger upwards, a none-too-subtle digital erection. The fig was so symbolic of erections that this gesture was known as 'giving the fig'. The custom survived into Roman times through the Dark Ages and spread across mediaeval Italy, Spain and France. The custom reached England in time for Shakespeare to include it in *Henry V*. It persists in modern times in the innocuous phrase 'I couldn't give a fig', and in the gesture of first resort for enraged drivers everywhere.

Whether or not the fig's aphrodisiac qualities extend beyond symbolism, tradition and sexual suggestion is moot. The fruit does contain an unusually high concentration of flavonoids, polyphenols and antioxidants which can help strengthen and prolong sexual desire. There is nothing, however, that marks figs out from other fruit with similar nutritional payloads but less salty reputations. The brain is the largest sexual organ so psychological triggers are certainly not to be sniffed at. Better to simply go with the flow, tuck into that splayed fig's juicy cavity and make like Cleopatra.

When it comes to enhancing the fig's seductive power it is hard to improve on nature. There are a few tips to bring out the fig's inner ooh-la-la. Ripeness is key to its sensuality and culinary possibility. Select oozing, soft to the touch, deep purple specimens from as good a source as you can find, preferably straight from the tree. Figs spoil very fast so are seldom good from a supermarket. To add a gourmet twist and bolster those aphrodisiac credentials you can inject the fruit with truffled honey to create a sensual, messy and utterly divine sex bomb. Serve as a starter or light lunch with salty goat's cheese and basil crostini – eat with your hands and keep a few tissues handy for later.

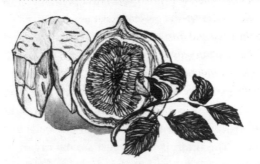

Honeyed Figs with Goat's Cheese and Purple Basil Crostini

Figs : 6
Truffle honey : 6 tsp
Ciabatta bread : 1 fresh loaf
Olive oil : 2 tbsp
Purple basil : a handful
Soft goat's cheese : 150 g
Salt and pepper : to taste

Truffle honey is available from good Italian delicatessens – if you can't find any, plain honey will suffice.

Cut the stalks from the figs and using a straw make a small hole through the top of each into the cavity of the fruit.

Warm the honey until it is very runny, then use the straw to suck it up and inject into each fig. Place the figs in a warming oven (80°C) for 5 minutes or on a sunny windowsill.

Heat a dry griddle pan.

Cut the ciabatta into six 1.5 cm thick slices. Dip each slice

in olive oil on both sides. Then pop into the pan to cook for 1
minute on each side until crisp and golden brown.

Roughly chop the basil and mix with the goat's cheese. Top
the crostini with the mix and season generously with salt and
pepper. Pop the crostini under the grill for a minute to brown
and serve immediately with the warm figs.

MANGO

In India the mango is massive. The tree can grant wishes, and
is a symbol of love, fertility and wealth. The leaves bring luck at
New Year and bless weddings with babies. The fruit is the food
of the gods. It can also feed more earthly appetites and is eulo-
gised in Ayurvedic texts as a potent aphrodisiac.

The mighty Mughal emperor Akbar was so impressed by
the mango that he planted the Lakhi Bagh, a grove of 100,000
mango trees. India is still the world's largest producer, growing
upwards of 13 million tonnes of mango a year – none of which
are exported. Some years back I accounted for a few kilos of this
gargantuan crop myself and had my own moment of mango
magic. One woodland wander in southern India I came across
a magnificent mango tree. It was the height of the mango
season and the tree was heavy with fruit. The air was heady with
sweet fragrance and hummed with insect energy. It seemed a
good place for a moment's repose. I picked up a fallen fruit,
split it open and bit into the amber flesh. Sticky juice ran from
my mouth whilst the floral sweetness intoxicated my refined
palate. Fruit after fruit I devoured, tossing the spent stones on

the ground. Saturated and sated with mango, I felt very good indeed, and wondered what I could do next. Fortunately my lady friend and no one else was near at hand.

In Ayurvedic medicine the body is believed to consist of seven elements: blood, bone, fat, plasma, marrow, flesh and sexual essence. Mangos nourish *shukra dhatu* (sexual essence), rejuvenating the male reproductive system and increasing the quality and quantity of semen. Mangos also feed *rakta dhatu* (blood), strengthening circulation. This boosts sexual energy and stamina, combating limp libido and wilting weenies. Mangos also get a mention in the Kama Sutra. This illustrious manual details the seven stages to flawless fellatio. The penultimate manoeuvre is coyly called *amrachushita* or 'sucking a mango fruit'. The description on how to master this ancient art is less coy: 'Take the penis deep into the mouth. Pull upon it and suck vigorously as though stripping clean a mango stone.' When mastered, sucking the mango fruit should be rapidly followed by the last hurrah of the all too obvious 'swallowing up' stage. Not much left to the imagination there.

Amrachushita and Ayurveda aside, the flesh of a perfectly ripe mango is a sensual delight, slithery smooth, softly yielding and slick with satin juice. The taste is a mouth-watering fusion of sweetness and subtle acidity. The mango's nutritional bounty of beta-carotene and vitamins C and E is responsible for its rich colour and addictive sharp–sweet flavour. It may also be responsible for the mango's aphrodisiac reputation. Boffins at Berkeley University in California conducted tests on ninety healthy men and found that those with diets rich in these three antioxidants had the highest sperm count and semen quality. Mangos are also rich in copper, a mineral necessary for the production of red blood cells and hence good circulation. All of which chimes rather pleasingly with the ancient Ayurvedic beliefs.

Should you wish to dance the nocturnal mango tango there are plenty of wonderful ways to prepare this fruit. On a hot day in the dusty subcontinent, nothing refreshes quite like a frothy mango lassi – simply whizz up fresh mango with yoghurt, honey and milk. Another classic complement is lime, which contrasts zingily with the sweetness of the mango. This can be eaten just so, or mix with avocado as a summery side to a dish of lime-cured salmon ceviche. If you want to up the aphrodisiac ante and really strut your stuff, make a fresh mango salsa and serve with steamed bok choi and caramelised scallops.

....

Mango Lassi

Fresh mango pulp : 150 g
Greek yoghurt . 150 g
Milk : 150 ml
Honey : 2 tsp (to taste)
Salt : a pinch

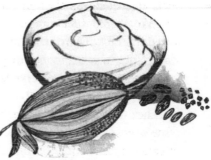

Select a very ripe mango whose skin springs to the touch. Slice either side of the central stone and scoop out the flesh with a spoon.

Place the yoghurt, mango and milk in a blender and whizz until smooth.

Add the honey and salt to taste.

Mango Salsa with Caramelised Scallops and Bok Choi

MANGO SALSA

Mango : 1 large ripe specimen

Ginger root : 1 cm

Coriander leaf : 1 handful

Spring onion : 2 large

Sweet chilli dipping sauce : 1 tbsp

Fish sauce : 1 tsp

Freshly squeezed lime juice : 1 tbsp

Black sesame seeds : 1 tsp

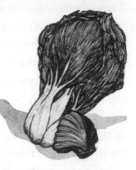

As before, slice vertically to either side of the thin stone and scoop the flesh from the skin with a spoon. This is a good test of ripeness. Dice the flesh into as near as you can to ½ cm-sized cubes.

Peel the ginger and chop the coriander as finely as possible. Thinly slice the spring onion on the diagonal.

Mix the spring onion, mango, ginger and coriander with the sweet chilli dipping sauce, fish sauce and lime juice. Stir thoroughly to combine and leave for the flavours to mingle. This can even be done the day before serving.

CARAMELISED SCALLOPS

Scallops : 6 fresh and fat king scallops (10 for a main course)

Sea salt : 100 g

Boiling water : 100 ml

Cold water : 400 ml

Vanilla extract : ½ tsp

Clarified butter : 2 tbsp

Flaky sea salt : a good pinch

The next step is to brine the scallops to intensify their flavour. In a bowl combine the salt and boiling water, and stir until the salt has dissolved. Add the cold water and the vanilla extract. Add the scallops to the brine and leave to soak for about 10 minutes.

Remove the scallops, rinse under cold water, pat dry with kitchen towel, cover and leave to relax in the fridge for 2 hours.

DRESSING

Bok choi : 2 heads
Light soy sauce : 1 tsp
Toasted sesame oil : 1 tsp
Rice vinegar : 1 tsp

Break the bok choi apart into separate leaves and steam for 3 minutes until lightly cooked.

Mix together the soy sauce, sesame oil and rice vinegar and add this dressing to the cooked bok choi. Allow the bok choi to cool in the dressing.

Heat 2 tablespoons of clarified butter in a heavy frying pan over a medium-high heat.

Season the scallops with a little flaky sea salt and place in the hot pan. After 3 minutes turn and cook the other side.

Serve the scallops in a line, each one on top of a small mound of mango salsa. Accompany with a heap of the dressed bok choi and sprinkle with black sesame seeds. Enjoy with a glass or two of chilled Alsace Gewürztraminer.

PINEAPPLE

Exotic and erotic, the pineapple has plenty to recommend itself to the foodie lover. Striking good looks, sweet, juicy and loaded with vitamins and enzymes, the pineapple has got it going on; and can probably get it going on for you too.

Christopher Columbus stumbled across the pineapple on his second voyage to the New World. In 1493 the expedition struck the coast of Guadalupe. The local Carib village greeted the pale-faced sea people with offerings of fresh pineapples. The pineapples impressed. Columbus shipped them back to Spain where they became an instant hit with the great and the good. At the most important banquets, pineapples had pride of place on the heaving tables of delicacies. At first only preserved pineapples were available to thrill their epicurean fans – the transatlantic crossing was too much for this sensitive fruit celebrity. Over the next centuries the enduringly expensive pineapple became a symbol of hospitality and largesse. It was a great honour to be treated to a pineapple-topped dinner display. The high cost, however, meant that the fruit was sometimes used purely for decoration as penny-pinching hosts would hire a pineapple for one night only – a glamorous fruity hostess to wow the guests.

The pineapple is not just a trophy. After dark it has the ability to perk up the most malingering of libidos. Manganese and vitamin C are key to keeping hormone levels sexy. A few slices of pineapple deliver the required daily doses. Bromelain provides pineapple with additional perkiness. This protein-digesting enzyme thins the blood, improves circulation and markedly improves disappointing pants-performance. The power of bromelain is also used commercially to tenderise tough meat – need we say more? Those interested in the after-hours oral arts will also be stirred to learn that pineapple is rather sweetening. Apparently effective on both sexes, pineapple delivers satisfied swallows all round – patrons of the oral arts should heartily applaud.

The gastronomic possibilities of the pineapple are far from endless. Its sour–sweet flavour is deliciously refreshing but difficult to combine with other ingredients. Lime-marinated chunks of fresh pineapple served with chilli gunpowder makes a refreshingly spicy cocktail snack. What better to nibble on when coolly sipping a coconut-water pina colada whilst savouring a tropical sunset? Let the meat tenderising and sweet swallowing begin.

PICKING YOUR PINEAPPLE

Once harvested, pineapples do not ripen any further. Unfortunately ripe pineapples do not last long. These two facts mean that most pineapples on Western shelves are not at their best. Make like an inquisitive hound, and sniff the indignant fruit's flat bottom. The pineapple's sweet aroma should penetrate the tough skin from here and here only. If the whole fruit smells the pineapple is overripe and has already started fermenting. If there is no fragrance at all the fruit is irredeemably underripe.

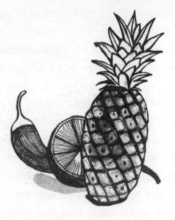

Pineapple with Chilli Gunpowder

Pineapple : 1
Lime : 1
Crushed black pepper : 1 tsp
Chilli powder (ancho if possible) : 1 tsp
Flaky sea salt : 1 tsp

*Skin and core your pineapple. Cut into bite-sized chunks and
squeeze the juice of one lime over the pineapple to marinate.*

*Crush the black pepper in a pestle and mortar and mix with a
medium to mild chilli powder and the flaky sea salt.*

*Serve the pineapple in a bowl with a small dish of chilli
gunpowder and dip away.*

Coconut-water Pina Colada

White rum : 50–100 ml

Pineapple juice : 100 ml

Coconut water : 100 ml

Ice : plenty

The bon viveur's take on the pina colada is clean and refreshing, substituting coconut cream with coconut water. Depending how boozy you like your beverages, measure out between two and four 25 ml shots of quality light rum. Shake the rum with the pineapple juice and coconut water. Serve over ice in a tumbler and garnish with a slice of pineapple and a slice of lime.

....

QUINCE

The belle of yesterday's ball, the quince is an overlooked and under-loved aphrodisiac. Not many people know that the original marmalade was made from stewed quince. Still fewer know that said marmalade was Tudor England's number one aphrodisiac. Look past the quince's pale knobbly skin, raw bitterness and grainy flesh. Focus instead on its heady floral aroma and sharp, sweet cooked flavour. The reputation may be a little wizened but the mythic golden apple still has the power to charm your pants off.

The quince is a distant cousin of apples and pears, and looks like a cross between the two. Cultivated long before apples were on the menu, it is most probably the object of ancient references to apples. The apple of desire that tempted Eve in the Garden of Eden was almost certainly a quince. In ancient Greece it was sacred to Aphrodite, the ravishing goddess of love and beauty. It was a ritual offering at weddings: at the end of the celebrations the bride would take a bite of the quince before entering the bridal chamber to join her new husband. It is easy to see how this pagan fertility ritual was hijacked in the tale of the Garden of Eden.

The nutritional foundation for quince's sinful reputation is surprisingly sturdy. The fruit's stand-out features are its delightful floral aroma and its extraordinarily high levels of pectin and plant mucilage. Quince's aromatic essential oil has been extracted since Roman times, and is a key ingredient in come-hither perfumes. It has the same aromatic chemicals as the musky pheromonal pong of truffles. Dimethyl disulphide has been scientifically shown to act as a feminine sexual pheromone in both lab rats and golden hamsters. Quince's high levels of mucilage, which is a sort of plant slime, are believed to aid the delightful slippery sliding of naturally lubricated love.

If you expect a ripe quince to have the texture and taste its nutritional properties suggest, you are in for a crunchy bitter surprise. Raw quince is extremely astringent and bitter. To unleash its charms it must be cooked and sweetened. The Greeks baked honey-filled quinces in pastry. The Romans discovered that stewing quince with honey resulted in a paste that set, the origin of all jams and marmalades. The granular texture of quince, even when stewed, is not ideal. To appreciate quince in all its sensuous glory, you need to strain its stewed paste through muslin. This is done to great culinary effect with membrillo, the classic Spanish sidekick to Manchego cheese. Slightly sweeter and less concentrated is quince jelly. Trembling on a crumpet at teatime or mixed through apple sauce for a porky Sunday lunch, it is delicious and well worth a few hours spent connecting with jam history.

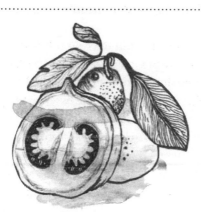

Quince Jelly
Quince : 1 kg
Sugar : 400 g

Remove the stems and cores from the quince and cut into quarters, leaving the skin on. Place in a pan and cover with water. Heat gently and stir until all the sugar is dissolved, then bring to the boil and simmer for an hour.

Using a masher, pulp the cooked quince into something that looks like a sloppy, rosy-coloured apple sauce. Add a little more water if the mixture is too thick.

Place the sauce in a colander lined with two layers of

cheesecloth and let the juice drip into a bowl leaving the pulp behind. This may take several hours.

You should get around 500 ml of quince juice from this process. Pour into a pan and add 400 g of sugar (the amount of sugar should be about 80 per cent the volume of juice). Bring to the boil gently, stirring constantly until the sugar has dissolved.

Place a jam thermometer into the jelly and skim off any foam that comes to the surface as it boils. Once the temperature reaches 105°C test the jelly by dripping a spoonful on to a cold plate. It should become sticky and tacky as it cools.

Pour the jelly into warmed and sterilised jars and screw on their lids while still hot. The heat will sterilise the headspace and as the jelly cools a vacuum will form which should keep the jelly good for years.

WATERMELON

Conspicuously large with brilliant red flesh, it is a little surprising that the watermelon's aphrodisiac oomph evaded detection until only a few years ago. Originating in the Kalahari of southern Africa, this supersized relative of the cucumber has been cultivated since ancient times. Travelling to the New World on slave ships, it was in the southern states of the USA that the watermelon was first fully appreciated.

Such disparate figures as gourmet president Thomas Jefferson and wild philosophic poet Henry Thoreau were enthusiastic propagators. Mark Twain hailed the watermelon as 'chief of this world's luxuries, king by grace of God over all fruits of the earth. When one has tasted it, he knows what the angels eat.' Whether or not this glowing reference is attributable to the watermelon's aphrodisiac qualities is unknown. Watermelon has traditionally had a thoroughly chaste reputation – a staple of summer holidays, BBQs and pool parties. This all changed when a team of scientists from Texas discovered that watermelon was actually Viagra in disguise. Overnight the watermelon grew up, left the playground and started hanging out in cool cocktail bars and fancy fusion restaurants.

The amino acid citrulline is responsible for this sudden change in status. Found in the flesh and rind of the watermelon, citrulline triggers the body to release arginine. When we get turned on arginine is metabolised to release nitric oxide, which dilates blood vessels causing the stiff nipples, sexual flush and bulging crotch of everyday arousal. In this instance more is definitely merrier. Put away half a watermelon and men may reach for the ruler, eager to record the statistics of their manly monolith.

The gastronomic possibilities of the watermelon are concise but none the worse for that. It shines au naturel but positively glows with an adult transfusion of rosé wine, vodka or tequila. In the kitchen, watermelon can be substituted effectively for its close cousin the cucumber. Try it with feta, olives, tomato and mint in a Greek salad with a difference. Better yet, use chunks in a deconstructed salad of aromatic duck, spring onion and deep-fried wontons, drizzled with a sweet soy dressing and scattered with toasted sesame seeds.

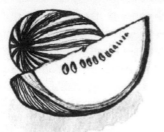

Margarita Watermelon

Watermelon : 1
Silver tequila : 200 ml
Triple Sec : 100 ml
Lime juice (1 large lime) : 50 ml
Sugar syrup : 50 ml

Select a modestly sized ripe watermelon. It should be heavy with juice and protest with a dull thud when thumped.

Prepare the margarita mix by simply stirring all the liquid ingredients together and sweetening with sugar syrup to taste. Those salty of spirit can skip the sugar altogether and season with sea salt.

Prepare the watermelon by making an incision around the stalk and cutting it out in one piece. Scoop out some flesh to make an internal chamber and fill this with the tequila mix. Replace the stalk plug to seal and leave to chill in the fridge for at least 3 hours.

If you are feeling the fiesta you can double-dose the watermelon, feeding it another ration of grog after a few hours,

*by which time the initial dousing will have distributed itself
throughout the flesh.*

*Serve the watermelon in slices at a BBQ. If you require a little
more refinement, cut the melon into balls and serve on cocktail
sticks out of a hollowed-out watermelon shell.*

Aromatic Duck and Watermelon Salad

Duck legs : 2

Salt : 1 tsp

Star anise : 2

Szechuan peppercorns : 1 tsp

Cloves : 5

Cinnamon : 1 stick

Ginger : 2 cm

Spring onion : 6

Rice wine : 3 tbsp

Honey : 1 tsp

Vegetable oil : 1 litre

Wonton wrappers : 4

Rocket and mizuna leaves : 2 large handfuls

Chicory (endive) : 1

Sweet basil : 1 small bunch

Mint : 1 small bunch

Watermelon : ¼ small watermelon

Toasted sesame seeds : 2 tsp

First rub the duck with salt, working it into the skin.

*Prepare the marinade by heating the spices then crushing
them roughly in a pestle and mortar. Combine with the*

freshly sliced ginger, three roughly chopped spring onions, rice wine and honey. Rub it into the duck and leave to marinate overnight.

Gently steam the duck in its marinade for 3 hours. Remove from the steamer, pat dry with kitchen towel and leave to air dry for half an hour.

Pour vegetable oil into a pan up to a third full and heat until hot. Deep-fry the duck for 5 minutes until the skin is crisp and brown. Remove the duck from the oil and place on some kitchen towel to absorb the excess.

Slice the wonton wrappers into 1 cm strips and deep-fry in the hot oil for 3 minutes until the strips are golden brown and very crispy. Again place on kitchen towel to dry.

PLUM SAUCE DRESSING

Mild red chilli : 1 tsp
Garlic : 2 cloves
Ginger : 2 cm
Yellow plums : 3
Rice wine : 2 tbsp
Rice vinegar : 1 tbsp
Toasted sesame oil : 1 tbsp
Salt : a good pinch

Prepare the dressing by removing the seeds from the chilli and finely chopping. Crush the garlic and chop the ginger. Remove the stones from the plums and cut into small pieces. Place all the ingredients in a saucepan and cook over a low heat for 20 minutes – if the sauce begins to dry out add a little water.

Liquidise the sauce in a blender and pass through a sieve. If it is too thick, add some more water to loosen it.

Prepare the salad by first washing the leaves, then slicing the chicory lengthways and roughly chopping the herbs.

Slice the remaining three spring onions lengthways as finely as you can. Cut the watermelon into thin slivers and shred the duck.

Toss the salad ingredients with the sesame seeds and crispy wonton skins and pile artfully on to two serving plates. Drizzle some dressing over each salad and serve immediately with a crisp Kiwi Sauvignon Blanc.

All Things Animal

CHEESE

It is well known that France is a nation of cheesy lovers. The legendary French libido and the nation's insatiable appetite for funky dairy products are strongly suggestive of aphrodisiac activity under the rind.

Actually, it is the Germans who are the true kaisers of *Käse*. Fritz chomps his way through 30 kg of cheese a year, enough to cause quite a stir in the lederhosen department. Cheese may not look or smell particularly sexy but its nutritional lunch-box positively pulses with aphrodisiac energy. Cheese not only boasts an all-star line-up of phenylethylamine (PEA), casein, histamine, tryptophan and magnesium but also sweetens the saliva to make ready for a spot of smooching.

Madly in love, sex-hungry couples feel that way because of PEA. It triggers the release of the pleasure-craving chemical dopamine. It is the main reason that chocolate is often held up to be an aphrodisiac (see Chocolate on page 213). Despite not usually being regarded as romantic, some varieties of cheese contain up to ten times as much PEA as chocolate. Although this chemical is metabolised quickly in the stomach, the levels in cheese are high enough to allow significant quantities to make their way to the brain and bring on that loving feeling. Allow a molten piece of oozing Brie to melt on your tongue and the chemicals can enter the bloodstream through the mouth's mucal membrane. The short distance from mouth to brain makes the likelihood of this active ingredient causing a commotion even greater.

Eighty per cent of the protein in cheese is a substance called casein. In the stomach casein is broken down into a natural opioid called casomorphin. As the name suggests this opoid is a cheesy cousin of morphine, quite capable of bringing on the same calming feelings of well-being and elation. It is a throwback to the original purpose of milk, namely nourishing a newborn. In order to bond baby to the nursing mother he or she is rewarded with a narcotic hit on every suckle. This calming opioid effect is enhanced by the action of tryptophan. Tryptophan is the essential amino acid that produces the hormonal harbinger of happiness, serotonin. The body is incapable of generating its own tryptophan so must rely on diet to get by. Fortunately mature cheeses, Parmesan in particular, are tryptophan treasure troves.

Tryptophan and casein would probably send one into a blissful snooze if they were not counteracted by the energising effect of histamine. Blue cheese and Parmesan both contain significant quantities of this unequivocal aphrodisiac. The sexual power of histamine is seen most clearly in its use as an extreme remedy for a drooping libido. A quick intravenous injection into the old man and he springs to attention. Elevated histamine levels are also consistent with a high sex drive and increased awareness. Released as part of sexual arousal, histamine triggers the telltale flush of feminine friskiness but more importantly enables and accelerates orgasm; both are in essence allergic biological responses to stimulation, chiming with histamine's other function as a controller of allergic reactions. One of the reasons sneezing is ever so slightly orgasmic.

The final piece of the aphrodisiac jigsaw is magnesium. Conspicuously lacking in the modern diet, magnesium is key to the production of sex hormones; I also hear whispers from my louche lady friends that it ushers in earth-shattering orgasms. The sea salts used in the manufacture of certain cheeses provide this mineral boost. The aphrodisiac Dunlop cheese from Islay in Scotland owes its naughty reputation to the unusually high magnesium levels in the local salt.

Despite this array of nutritional evidence, as an aphrodisiac cheese has limited historical pedigree. Milk, however, enjoys ageless endorsement. The Arab world is agog with the stimulating properties of camel's milk, whilst Indian bridegrooms fight first-night nerves with a restorative draught of milk and almonds spiced with pepper. As it is essentially concentrated milk, I think it fair to add these milky attributes to the cheese tally. One main reason there is limited cheese history is because modern cheese-making only really took off in the Middle Ages. The original blue cheese, Roquefort, developed an aphrodisiac reputation almost immediately and it was honoured with a royal patent in the thirteenth century. Casanova added his own age-inclusive, off-colour endorsement, commending it as a sure-fire way to both 'restore an old love and ripen a young one'.

When selecting suitable cheeses to adorn the aphrodisiac board one is spoilt for choice. Like a triumphant tumble, a good cheeseboard should provide softness, hardness and a little bit of blue. The Italian threesome of oozing Burrata, salty crystalline Parmigiano-Reggiano and creamy blue Gorgonzola should do the trick. Serve with grapes, some exceptional bread and lots of red wine. If you want to flex your culinary muscles and instigate an orgy, serve up fondue. This oozy molten mess is the stairway to cheese heaven. *Fondue Piémontaise* is made with

Fontina cheese emboldened with butter, egg yolk and chopped white truffles. Delightful but ditched at the altar for the incomparable *Fondue Normande* – a dish I would happily marry.

Fondue Normande

Garlic : 1 clove
Pont-L'Évêque : 100 g
Camembert : 100 g
Livarot : 100 g
Cornflour : 1 tbsp
Dry cider : 100 ml
Calvados : 75 ml
Salt and pepper : to taste

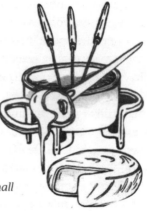

Cut the garlic clove in half and rub vigorously around the inside of a small copper pan or fondue dish.

Trim the rind from the three cheeses, cut them into small pieces and place in the pan.

Mix the cornflour with the cider and pour over the cheese.

Gently heat the pan, stirring all the time. Once the cheese has melted and combined with the cider increase the heat to around 90°C to cook out the cornflour. Do not let the fondue boil.

Season with salt and pepper then add the Calvados.

Place the pan on the dining table over a spirit burner and serve with plenty of bread.

Get dunking.

EGGS

No self-respecting breakfast leaves the kitchen without two eggs on the plate. Poached, scrambled, boiled or baked, sunnyside up or overeasy, eggs are the most versatile of ingredients. Enjoyed by man since monkey times, the egg's association with fertility and potency are almost as ancient.

An egg is a wonder – a seemingly inanimate object from which new life spontaneously springs. It makes perfect sense that our ancestors believed they could absorb this magic with a hearty cooked breakfast. The advent of science has demystified but not discredited this mini-miracle. An egg is a self-sufficient store of everything an embryo needs to develop and grow, an incredible concentration of energy, protein and vital nutrients. Understandably, this rich cocktail is quite the tonic for those with reproductionary recreation on their mind.

In ancient Greece, the sparrow was sacred to the love goddess Aphrodite. Sparrow eggs were the most prized of all aphrodisiacs. This belief spread to India with Alexander and was firmly established when the Kama Sutra was written. Those eager to enjoy many women are exhorted to drink deep of a boiled mix of 'rice and eggs of sparrow with milk, ghee and honey'. In Central America and South-East Asia the aphrodisiac hammer falls upon the unfortunate turtle: the passion for its libido-loosening eggs drives an illicit trade that augurs ill for the survival of the species. Sparrow and turtle eggs may seem a little outlandish but they are nothing compared with the Balut egg aphrodisiac of the Philippines. This is a fertilised and incubated duck egg that rewards the intrepid gastronaut with a meaty egg and the crispy crunch of bone and beak.

Refined and defiantly eccentric, the English upper class may swear by gulls' eggs, but for the average Joe it is the chicken that provides the everyday egg. Domesticated in the East, the chicken did not reach Western Europe until the fifth century BC and didn't reach America until Columbus took it there in the fifteenth century. Making up for lost time, the world now gobbles up over one trillion hen's eggs a year.

Hen's eggs provide an astonishingly rich nutritional package. I attribute their aphrodisiac efficiency to an unusual and well-balanced bonanza of essential fatty acids. I eulogise elsewhere about the loving effects of tryptophan, lysine, tyrosine, histidine and arginine. The two-egg breakfast provides them all in abundant quantity, more than enough to keep eyes bright, tails bushy and libidos wagging appreciatively.

In gastronomy the egg gets around, not only a principal ingredient in innumerable dishes but an elemental building block in baking, patisserie, pasta and desserts. The taste of an egg will vary according to its freshness and the diet of the mother hen. Every egg in addition to the white and yolk has an air sac under the shell. As the egg ages moisture evaporates, enlarging this air space. If suspicious of your egg's suitability for an aphrodisiac encounter, drop it into 500 ml of water mixed with 60 g of salt. A fantastically fresh egg will sink, an acceptable egg hovers halfway, whilst the bad egg floats at the surface.

When poaching, the fresh egg is your friend. The gelatinous white clings tightly to the yolk. Poached eggs make admirable brunch dishes coupled with aspagarus or bathed in hollandaise for eggs Benedict. However, to wring out every sensuous drop you simply have to scramble. Serve scattered with chopped anchovy and parsley on a roast field mushroom sitting on a square of fried bread. Egg perfection matched only by the pocket-sized marvel of *oeufs en cocotte*. These baked beauties are elegant enough to kick off the most refined dinner party – simply top with caviar or match with smoked haddock and a dusting of Parmesan.

....

Scrambled Eggs with Roast Field Mushroom
Field mushrooms : 2
Salt and pepper : to taste
Butter : 50 g
Eggs : 4
Milk : 2 tbsp
Wholegrain bread : 2 slices
Salted anchovy : 2 fillets
Parsley : 1 sprig

Preheat the oven to 170°C.
First select two very
large field mushrooms or Portobello
mushrooms. Remove the stalk from each and
season with salt and pepper. Place a knob of butter on each and
roast in the oven for 30 minutes, basting every so often.
When it comes to making scrambled egg, success is in the
detail. The pan must be non-stick (or extremely well seasoned)
with a heavy base to keep an even temperature. The eggs must
be fresh and the heat must be feeble.

Crack the eggs into a jug and add the milk. With a fork whisk the eggs enough to combine thoroughly but not so much as to aerate the egg mix.

Slice two thick pieces of wholegrain bread, remove the crusts and fry in half the remaining butter until golden brown on both sides.

Rinse the anchovy fillets of excess salt then finely chop.

Strip the parsley from the stem and again chop finely.

Place the remaining butter in your carefully selected non-stick pan and heat moderately until the butter has melted. When it begins to foam pour in your egg mix and reduce to a low heat.

The initial heat will thicken the bottom layer of egg very quickly; gently dislodge this from the base of the pan so it remains in largeish pieces. Continue with this process of allowing a layer of egg to half-form then dislodging it until the scrambled egg is almost ready. Remove from the heat as the residual temperature in the pan will finish the cooking.

Place one square of fried bread in the centre of the serving plate. Top with a baked mushroom and fill the mushroom with a pile of scrambled egg. Sprinkle the scrambled egg with chopped anchovy and parsley then season with freshly ground pepper.

If you want to turn this into a more formal brunch or supper dish serve with dressed lamb's leaf lettuce around the mushroom.

Smoked Haddock *Oeufs en Cocotte*

Milk : 200 ml
Bay leaf : 1
Peppercorns : 3
Smoked haddock : 100 g
Butter : for greasing
Heavy double cream : 60 ml
Eggs : 2
Grated Parmesan : 2 tbsp
Salt and pepper : to taste

Preheat the oven to 200°C.

Heat the milk in a pan with the bay leaf and peppercorns. Bring the milk to a light simmer and allow the flavours to infuse for 5 minutes. Place the haddock into the milk and remove from the heat. The fish will cook as the milk cools. Once the milk is tepid remove the fish and flake, discarding the skin.

Butter two ramekins or cocotte pots. Spoon 1 tablespoon of cream into each ramekin and cover with flaked haddock.

Crack a very large egg into each ramekin, spoon 2 more tablespoons of cream over the egg and cook in a bain-marie in the oven for 10 – 12 minutes.

Remove the eggs from the oven, season with black pepper and sea salt, then sprinkle with the grated Parmesan. Serve immediately with some crusty white bread.

FOIE GRAS

Like mink coats, caviar and champagne, foie gras is a byword for luxury. It is firmly established in the international jet set. If there were such a thing as a gastronomic VIP area, that is where foie gras would be, hobnobbing with aristocrats, oligarchs, beautiful women and Botox. Rich, delicate flavour and satin texture are sensual delights but it is the whiff of power, money and glamour that makes foie gras such a potent aphrodisiac. It's the law of the jungle; high status means more mating. In our sophisticated world what better way for a bon viveur to signal such status than a foie gras stuffing?

For all its glamour, foie gras has pretty seamy origins. The blood diamond of the kitchen, every buttery bite gives the karma a battering. Foie gras means 'fat liver', but refers specifically to goose liver. Duck foie gras, the only other variant, is similar but less rich. Farmers create these 'fat livers' with a strict diet of far too much food, far too often. As ducks and geese naturally like to watch their weight, these mega meals are unceremoniously force-fed into the protesting fowl using a metal pipe. The excess energy is stored as fat in these waterfowls' livers – an evolutionary quirk ruthlessly exploited to produce livers around ten times their natural size.

This bizarre culinary practice was established a bewilderingly long time ago. Around 2500 BC, the Egyptians discovered that forced over-feeding resulted in fattened geese. The Romans, true to decadent form, developed the technique further, using dried figs to create geese with gargantuan livers. Pliny the Elder attributes this gluttonous breakthrough to the gastronome

Marcus Gavius Apicius, a man he admiringly describes as 'born to enjoy every extravagant luxury that could be contrived':

Apicius made the discovery, that we may employ the same artificial method of increasing the size of the liver of the sow, as of that of the goose; it consists in cramming them with dried figs, and when they are fat enough, they are drenched with wine mixed with honey, and immediately killed

With the decline and fall of the Roman Empire, it fell to the Jews to preserve this ancient technique through the Dark Ages. The gastronomic awakening of eighteenth-century France saw foie gras reborn and clasped to the nation's bosom. South-west France is now the centre of world production, churning out almost 20,000 tonnes of fatty liver a year.

Interest piqued, a few years ago I paid a visit to a foie gras farm in the Périgord. I am pleased to report that modern production is not as barbarous as perhaps it sounds. The force-feeding takes place only for the last fortnight of the bird's life, and to the bon viveur's untrained eye it almost looked as though they were enjoying the process. They were certainly queuing up at feeding time. Guilt partially assuaged, I procured a lobe of the finest liver and retired to the chateau to investigate its preparation.

Cooking with fresh foie gras needs a delicate touch. One can watch with horror as the prized delicacy dissolves in a hot pan. Half-freezing before use and brushing with honey gives you time to sear a slice in a hot pan without it melting away. The honey helps caramelise the foie gras slice, creating a crisp crust with an oozing soft centre. This is traditionally placed on top of a fillet steak, but I prefer a lighter partner. The balance is perfect with a fat fillet of roast cod. Hot foie gras is fantastic but it is more usual to serve it chilled as a terrine. Preparing a terrine is far less prone to error. The liver needs to be marinated overnight and can then be baked in a bain-marie, poached in fat or water, steamed or simply cured in salt. The cooked foie gras needs to be well refrigerated before serving, to allow the sublimely smooth buttery texture to fully develop. The richness of the foie gras is usually contrasted with a sharp fruity accompaniment and toast. After maximum enjoyment with minimum aggravation, I would dazzle a dining companion with a robustly flavoured duck foie gras, cured in salt, served with toasted walnut bread and sour plum caramel.

Salt-Cured Duck Foie Gras with Mirabelle and Sour Plum Caramel

Raw duck foie gras : 250 g
Mirabelle or Armagnac : 1 tbsp
Sea salt : a pinch
Black pepper : 1 large pinch
Coarse-grained salt : 1 kg
Granulated sugar : 250 g + 50g
Greengages or plums : 4
Red wine vinegar : 2 tbsp

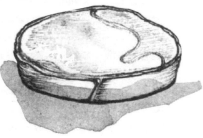

If your foie gras hasn't been cleaned and deveined this is a task you must perform. Unwrap your pale beige liver, trim off any yellowy green spots and pull away any white membrane clinging

to the outside. Unfold the two lobes of the liver and gently pull them apart. They are connected by a vein into the centre of each lobe. Cut this and with tweezers gently tease it out from each lobe with a slow even motion. It all happens a lot easier if the liver is at room temperature.

Lay the lobes of foie gras out on a sheet of greaseproof paper, sprinkle with the Mirabelle eau de vie or Armagnac and season with a little sea salt and pepper. Roll the foie gras into a tight cylinder about 6 cm in diameter and tie off both ends. Refrigerate for 1 hour.

Remove the greaseproof paper and wrap the foie gras in one layer of cheesecloth. Tie each end and shape so it forms a tight cylinder. Place the foie gras sausage in a suitable container and completely bury in a mix of 4 parts coarse-grained salt to 1 part granulated sugar. Refrigerate for 12 hours.

Remove the foie gras sausage from the salt, unwrap the cheesecloth and wrap in cling film for later.

Cut the greengages or plums in half lengthways and extract the stones. Slice into thin strips.

In a small pan mix 50 g of sugar with enough water for it to resemble wet sand. Cook over a low heat until the sugar turns a rich golden brown. Remove from the heat and add 2 tablespoons of red wine vinegar. Return to the heat and bring to the boil, stirring to combine. Add a good pinch of freshly ground black pepper and stir in the plum slices. Allow the mix to cool.

Serve a thick slice of foie gras sprinkled with a few grains of sea salt, accompanied by thin slices of walnut bread toast and an artful dollop of the sour plum caramel.

Seared Duck Foie Gras with Roast Cod

Cod fillets : 2
Melted butter : 1 tbsp
Honey : 1 tbsp
Raw duck foie gras : 2 slices
Plain flour : 1 tsp
Salt and pepper : to taste
Spinach : 2 large handfuls

Place an oiled roasting dish in an oven heated to 190°C. When the dish is hot add the cod fillets skin side down and brush with butter. Bake for 15 minutes. The cod is ready when a skewer can be inserted into the fish without meeting any resistance.

Meanwhile warm the honey to make it more liquid, brush the raw foie gras with it, toss in flour then season with salt and pepper.

Heat a non-stick frying pan to a medium-high heat. Sear the foie gras slices for about 30 seconds on each side, until a brown crust forms. Remove and keep warm while you quickly wilt the spinach in the same pan using the foie gras fat to coat. Season well.

Place a mound of spinach on each plate, remove the roast cod and place on top. Perch the seared foie gras on the cod fillet and serve with a side order of potato gratin.

HONEY

For thousands of years honey had a monopoly on sweetness. In our sugar-coated times it is hard to fully appreciate the honey buzz enjoyed by our ancestors.

Bees and honey inspired almost religious reverence. Honey was the food of the gods, a precious substance reserved for ritual and romance. The ancient Egyptians believed that bees were the tears of the sun god Ra. They offered honey to the fertility god Min to sweeten their lovemaking. Famously fond of oral sex, Cleopatra would honey her pot in preparation for the nightly onslaught. This may have been partially precautionary. Honey was also considered anti-bacterial and contraceptive, and she did get around.

Arabic gentlemen stuck in a sexual rut were prescribed honey mixed with ginger and pepper by the great eleventh-century physician Avicenna. Alternatively they could consult the legendary Arab sex manual, *The Perfumed Garden*. This erotic encyclopaedia commends honey, almonds and pine nuts to its randy readers. The Celtic and Viking barbarians preferred their honey alcoholic. Newly wed couples would kick-start conjugal bliss with a month tippling on honey wine – the origin of the modern-day honeymoon.

Honey production is unique. During the warm summer months, battalions of worker bees harvest flower nectar from the surrounding countryside. Back in the hive, teams repeatedly swallow and regurgitate the nectar until it is half-digested and halfway to honey. The final process is driving off the excess moisture to stop the honey going bad. Fanning their wings the bees turn the hive into an insect drying machine, concentrating the honey so it can be safely stored.

These days honey is more buttered crumpet than sticky strumpet. The aphrodisiac effect, however, remains intact. Honey is pure natural sugar. Evolution has hard-wired the human body to seek out such advantageous, energy-dense sweet foods. As a result sweetness now triggers the brain to release natural opiates and dopamine, spreading good feelings and the desire to seek out more sweetness in the future. Sex does exactly the same thing so it is quite natural that the two get amorously entwined in the mind. The problem is that sugar is now everywhere and in everything. Like addled addicts we have become accustomed to intense hits of sweetness. The drug no longer works. The spoonful of honey that would have triggered a tidal wave of sexually inspiring dopamine and opiate pleasure, today might just cause a ripple.

Although nutritionally diminished, honey remains the most gastronomically rewarding source of sweetness. The heady floral bouquet and perfumed sweetness of a pure honey add a sweet sensuality not found in sugar. Heather honey dribbled over Greek yoghurt, fresh raspberries and toasted oats is surely the summer breakfast of sex gods. Still better, retreat from the heat and submit to the chilly kiss of a honey, lemon and ginger sorbet served in a pool of iced honey vodka.

Honey, Lemon and Ginger Sorbet with Honey Vodka

Honey : 125 ml
Water : 600 ml
Lemon : ½ large lemon (unwaxed)
Ginger root : 3 cm length
Vodka : 50 ml

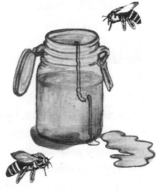

*Add 100 ml of honey and all of the
water to a saucepan. Thin, fine acacia
honey works particularly well in this
recipe but any honey will suffice.*

*Squeeze the juice from the lemon
and grate the zest. Peel and grate the ginger.*

*Add the ginger, lemon juice and zest to the pan and heat.
Bring to the boil and simmer for 1 minute.*

*Strain the mixture through a sieve. Taste and add further
lemon juice if more sharpness is required.*

*Transfer the mix into a container and when cool place in the
freezer (or ice-cream maker).*

*Once the sorbet has begun to freeze (after about two hours),
remove from the container and whizz up in a food processor
or blender. Return to the container and refreeze, repeating the
process after another hour. The finished sorbet should have a
consistency similar to crystallised honey.*

*To make the honey vodka, simply warm the vodka with the
remaining honey until it dissolves, then place in the freezer to
chill.*

To serve, pour one shot of syrupy vodka into the bottom of a

Martini glass or champagne coupe. Top with a generous scoop of sorbet.

....

IGUANA

The cuddly koala and scaly iguana do not have a lot in common. It is only upon intimate examination that a startling and most unusual similarity is revealed. Uniquely in the animal kingdom, both creatures sport a double penis. Appendages as impressive as these do not go unnoticed. Traditional communities throughout Central America duly revere the iguana as a paragon of virility. Unfortunately for iguanas, these communities also believe this celebrated potency is readily transferable through the medium of soup.

In Nicaragua during Holy Week, there is a veritable frenzy of iguana feasting. The Nicaraguans seek out bloated females, remove their cargo of unlaid eggs, and gleefully turn them into steaming bowls of iggy stew and hard-boiled iggy eggs. This primes the population for long nights of post-Lenten passion, and a noted national spike in births nine months later. The sexual prowess of the iguana has also been documented much closer to home. Mozart, a captive reptile in Antwerp zoo, heroically maintained an erection for over a week. Following a cold-blooded night of passion with no fewer than three licentious lady lizards (Truus, Pepina and Bianca), Mozart's ardour would not subside. Regrettably, fearing infection, vets were forced to amputate. Luckily, Mozart had a fully functioning spare to fall back on.

In certain circles, it is believed that a hearty bowl of iguana stew can cure impotence – a bold claim that needs more than a double penis to be taken seriously. Unsurprisingly, there is little direct research on the subject. However, as the iguana becomes an increasingly popular pet, there are a growing number of PhD theses documenting iguana biology. A cursory inspection immediately highlights the presence of a series of strange glands along the inner thigh of the iguana, glands which ooze a powerful sex pheromone during the mating season. Study into these secretions has shown a whole chromatograph of obscure fatty acids, all very rich in vitamin D. Production of our own sex hormones is extremely dependent on vitamin D, so it seems that soup infused with a healthy dose of iguana musk could well have a telling effect on the Central American libido.

Outside the jungle, procuring iguana poses problems. However, should an itinerant iguana just happen to come one's way, seize the opportunity with both hands (preferably just behind the neck). Lay on a stout final feed of beaten egg and brandy. Lower the lights, put a little Chopin on the gramophone and when the unfortunate beast is serenely slumbering apply the *coup de grâce*. A quick strike to the neck with a heavy cleaver should suffice – maximum decapitation with the minimum gore and personal disquiet. It is indeed rare that I would consider such a tortuous and morally ambiguous route to a meal, but if its many supporters are to be believed this is a palaver well worth the aggravation.

Although the most common iguana preparation is a soupy stew, I would advise against and plump for roast iguana. Genuinely tasty, roast iguana has a flavour and texture similar to chicken, but with more savoury notes. Unusually, iguana needs to be parboiled before roasting. In order to enhance the aphrodisiac qualities I would suggest that this is done with the skin on, to infuse the dish with seductive iguana secretions.

. . . .

Roast Iguana with Chipotle and Oregano Marinade

Iguana : 1 medium-sized specimen

Bay leaves : 3

Peppercorns : 2

Chipotle chilli : 2 dried chillies

Garlic : 4 fat cloves

Rice vinegar : 3 tbsp

Chopped oregano : 2 tbsp

Onion : 1 medium red onion

Vegetable oil : 1 tbsp

Tomatoes : 4

Coriander : 1 tbsp

Salt and pepper : to taste

Gound paprika : 1 tsp

Ground cinnamon : 1 tsp

Remove the innards from your iguana, retaining the heart. Cut off the head and split the body in two down the spine.

Place the iguana in a pot and cover with water. Add a few bay leaves and a couple of peppercorns, bring to the boil and simmer for 15 minutes.

Remove the iguana from the pot, reserving the poaching liquid. Allow the meat to cool and remove the skin. Cut the skinned iguana into pieces and place in a bowl ready to be marinated.

For the marinade, rehydrate the dried chillies and blend with two cloves of garlic, the vinegar and oregano to form a smooth paste. Add the paste to the meat, mix and leave to marinate for about 2 hours.

Place the marinated meat in a hot oven (220°C) and roast for about 45 minutes until tender. The exact time will depend on the size of your pieces of iguana.

While the iguana is roasting, prepare the sauce. Finely chop the onion and sweat for 10 minutes in a pan with a little oil and any remaining marinade, crush the remaining garlic and add to cook out for a couple of minutes.

Roughly chop the tomatoes and add the reserved poaching liquid to the pan. Bring to the boil and reduce until the sauce is the consistency of double cream.

Remove the sauce from the heat, add the chopped coriander and season with salt and pepper.

To serve, place a heap of cooked rice on the plate, ladle over lots of sauce and place the roast iguana on top. Squeeze a little lime over the meat and lightly dust with ground paprika and cinnamon.

STEAK

Call me a lion, but tearing into a piece of red meat makes me want to roar. Eating other animals has been the key to our evolution as terrestrial top dog. Sexual selection favours the successful hunter, and nothing prompts the hunting hero to select sex more than the carnivorous afterglow of a prime beefsteak. The blood is up, some dormant instinct stirs and the dressing gown of civilisation slips to the floor. The ancient inheritance awakes and the primal urge to procreate is on the prowl.

The cave paintings of Lascaux show that bovine beasties have been on the menu since prehistoric times. The French may splutter and the Americans mutter but it is the English who are responsible for the modern-day steak. The *Rosbifs* of the eighteenth century started the unstoppable trend for grilling individual slabs of prime beef: the Sublime Society of Beefsteaks' inauguration in 1735 bears testament to the entrenched English enthusiasm for grilled beef. It wasn't until Napoleon met his Waterloo in 1815 that steak was popularised on mainland Europe. The chefs of Paris picked up the habit catering for the red-blooded appetites of the British Army. Like a greasy English thumbprint on the white tablecloth of French gastronomy, the habit has stuck.

Whilst not strictly speaking an aphrodisiac tradition, it has long been believed that eating meat rich with blood bestows manly vim and vigour. In *Henry V*, Shakespeare describes poultry-loving French lords chickening out at the thought of the English soldiers who fight like devils after 'great meals of beef'. The belief was government policy by the eighteenth century, with each able-bodied seaman in the British Navy rationed a gut-busting 209 pounds (95 kg) of beef per year – equivalent to a 9-ounce steak every day.

Father of psychology Sigmund Freud was the first to link sex and aggression as the primary motivating forces in human behaviour. Modern nutrition shows that the sex hormone testosterone lies at the heart of both impulses. It also reveals that a slap-up feed of beef will not only boost testosterone but will provide a hit of libido-enlivening amino acids and minerals at the same time.

A moderate-sized steak provides more than the recommended daily dose of zinc and iron. A deficiency in either of these two minerals is strongly correlated to low libido and sexual malfunction in both men and women. The amino acids stirring the pot are tyrosine and arginine. Tyrosine is essential in the production of both dopamine and epiphedrine (adrenaline) – neurotransmitters connected to sex and aggression, and perhaps responsible for the murky link between the two. Arginine is more of a lover than a fighter, boosting the body's nitric oxide levels. Nitric oxide is something of a sexual superhero: lord of the trouser-tent and irrigator extraordinaire of the female forest.

Like all ostensibly simple things, cooking a steak well is surprisingly difficult. First off you need to have a good relationship with your butcher. Cajole him into releasing his finest dry-aged slab into your grateful hands. My general preference is for bone-in rib steak, aka the fabulous *côte de boeuf*. However, as two is the magic number for most affairs of the heart, I will focus on the shared pleasures of the porterhouse T-bone. Prepare it *alla*

Fiorentina with a rocket salad and bottle of Chianti on the side. There is only one better way to spend time with your loved one, and you can do that immediately afterwards.

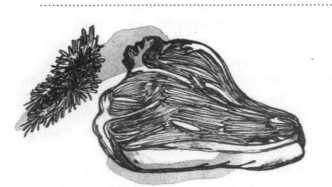

Bistecca alla Fiorentina

Porterhouse T-bone steak : 1
Rock salt : Lots
Rosemary : 4 large sprigs
Balsamic vinegar : 75 ml
Extra virgin olive oil : 75 ml
Lemon : 1
Rocket : 100 g
Charcoal, wood fire or griddle pan : 1
Sea salt and pepper : to taste

This recipe needs some advance planning as the curing and marinating process takes over 5 hours. First select a dry-aged steak of prime beef. It should be about 4 cm thick, well marbled (with fat distributed evenly throughout the meat) and dry to the touch. Stick to a quality butcher as supermarkets rarely sell dry-aged meat. If you want to go authentic, track down some Chianina beef, which comes from the massive white oxen reared in Tuscany and Umbria in Italy.

Place the steak on a bed of rock salt and cover in more rock salt. Leave for 2 hours. Remove the steaks from the salt, rinse with water and pat dry with a clean kitchen towel.

Roughly chop the rosemary and press into each side of the steak. Mix the balsamic vinegar and olive oil and pour over your steak. The dish really benefits from a top-quality balsamic vinegar so go with the best you can afford.

Leave the steak for 3 hours, turning once or twice.

Remove the steak from the marinade. Reserve both the marinade and the rosemary.

The fire to cook the meat on should be hot, but the flames should have died a little. Set the grill over the fire at a height where you can hold your hand for barely a couple of seconds because it is so hot. If you are indoors use a heavy cast-iron griddle pan – lightly oiled and heated until it is very hot.

Pat the steak with paper towel to ensure it is totally dry. Throw half the rosemary on to the fire (or into the griddle pan) and place the steak on the hot grill to sear in the fragrant smoke. After a couple of minutes the steak should come easily off the grill; flip it on to the uncooked side, throw on the remaining rosemary and season the cooked side with sea salt and pepper.

Once the second side is seared, raise the grill a little to slightly reduce the heat and continue flipping and seasoning the steak every couple of minutes until it is done. On a fire, rare

*should take about 16 minutes, medium-rare should take about
20 minutes. If you are using a griddle pan the steak will cook
quicker – reduce the cooking time by about 5 minutes.*

*Remove the steak from the fire and loosely cover in foil. Leave
to rest for half the cooking time, then cut the tenderloin and loin
steaks away from the T-bone. Carve into thick slices.*

*Present on a large wooden board with the cut meat fanning
out from the T-bone and serve with lemon wedges and a large
pile of rocket dressed in the reserved marinade.*

When rare steak just isn't raw enough, there is only one way
to go. Steak tartare is sushi for the steak lover. Minced cuts of
the best beef served mooing on the plate. If that doesn't unleash primal urges nothing will. There are as many recipes for
steak tartare as there are those who eat it. The classic version
seasons the beef (or sometimes horse) with capers, Worcester-
shire sauce, shallot, gherkins and mustard, serving it with a raw
egg yolk. The bon viveur's version is something of a departure,
dispensing with the raw egg yolk and replacing it with the olé
of peppery 100 per cent agave silver tequila and the sizzle of a
seared crust. This cooked style is known in France as 'aller-retour',
and in the USA as 'black and blue' – charred on the outside and
raw in the middle. Serve with melba toast and sliced avocado.

Agave Steak Tartare served 'Black and Blue'

Dry-aged fillet steak : 400 g

Silver tequila : 2 tbsp

Lime juice : 1 tbsp

Fish sauce : 1 tbsp

Black pepper : ½ tsp

Tabasco : 2 tsp

Coriander : a small bunch

Shallot : 1 medium shallot

Green jalapeños : 1 tbsp

Semi-dried tomatoes : 1 tbsp

Vegetable oil : 1 tbsp

Using a very sharp knife cut the beef into thin slices, then cut each slice into tiny cubes of meat. Place in a metal bowl and add the 100 per cent agave silver tequila, freshly squeezed lime juice, fish sauce, ground black pepper and Tabasco. Refrigerate for 2 hours.

Chop the coriander, shallot, green jalapeños and semi-dried tomatoes as fine as you can, keeping them separate.

Press the marinated meat into a 6 cm chef's ring or pastry cutter, then turn out to form two tall patties. Place in the freezer for 15 minutes to firm up.

Heat the oil in a heavy frying pan. When it begins to smoke and is incredibly hot, place the steaks in the pan. Fry for 5 seconds on each side.

Roll the seared steaks in the chopped coriander and serve

with petite heaps of the jalapeño, semi-dried tomato and
shallots for seasoning as you eat.

....

VENISON

The culinary call of the wild, venison is the most ancient and widely eaten game meat. Deer have sustained our development from none too civilised cavemen into the modern age. These mighty beasts' noble bearing, impressive antlers and lusty libido make their meat pure machismo. Venison has a mythic reputation: a testosterone-boosting superfood to power heroic feats of moonlit mating and general manliness.

The best venison comes from the red deer, monarch of the Scottish glens and emperor of the ancient English forest. Armed with a hip-flask of home-made plum gin, I set out one dewy autumn evening to witness an emperor at work. In darkest Suffolk with only a lanky landowning lord for company I stealthily approached a stag and his harem of ladies. The night was calm, punctuated by the occasional owlish hoot and squawk of roosting pheasants. Then the roaring began. Our emperor let rip with a guttural bellow of pure animal lust. The sound of the rut reverberated through the wooded valley as this king of forest set about his entourage, mounting and mating with impressive stamina.

Deer mate every autumn with a furious frenzy of pent-up sexuality. This feast of fornication is known as the rut. Every stag's diary is block-booked for this seminal event. A dominant stag will gather a harem of up to twenty hinds, and defend his mating rights to the death. The nightly bouts of sex and fighting last for about a month. At the end the stag is a shadow of his former self, having lost as much as 20 per cent of his body weight. Understandably, mankind is mightily impressed by this dedicated show of virility. The Lakota tribe of North America revered the elk as a symbol of strength, courage and sexual prowess. Rather less respectful to their fellow creatures, orgy-fatigued Romans sought to acquire the deer's sexual stamina by eating its penis. Hippocrates, the godfather of modern medicine, was the first to identify deer ding-a-ling as an aphrodisiac, way back in the fourth century BC. An ancient treatment for a timeless concern, it enjoys continued support in modern-day China. To maximise its medicinal properties the Chinese believe that the penis should be extracted from a wild stag while still alive. The uprooted organ is then steeped in alcohol to create the aphrodisiac deer-penis wine. All of which sounds jolly painful for the poor deer.

Painful and pointless, in fact. To date the active ingredient in deer penis has resolutely eluded nutritional research. Venison, however, provides much the same aphrodisiac goodness as top-quality beef. It boasts a balanced array of libido-boosting amino acids, zinc, iron and B vitamins. A low-fat, high-protein diet has been shown to stimulate testosterone production, and there are few meats as lean or as high in protein as venison. Psychologically there is a frisson about the flesh of an untamed animal. Canines cutting into hunks of venison invoke an ancient heritage, hunters returning victorious from the wilds, meat-filled bellies and primeval fireside tumblings.

Ethically, nutritionally and gastronomically it is best to pass on penis. The choice cuts of venison are fillet, haunch and liver. The taste and texture of venison is similar to beef but leaner, softer and with a distinct gamey taste. In the kitchen, venison also behaves very much like beef. Joints should be roasted, steaks grilled and liver pan-fried. The strong gamey flavour loves red wine, flourishes with a little bit of redcurrant sweetness and partners perfectly with the aromatic notes of juniper. The surprisingly mild liver is very much a hunter's treat, rarely reaching the butcher's counter. If you do come across some, dust in flour seasoned with ground juniper, pan-fry in clarified butter and serve with a reduction of redcurrant and red wine. Roast haunch of red deer is fit for a royal banquet. If your feast is for two, you may have to downsize to roe deer or even the diminutive muntjac. You will still have too much meat but that is the very essence of feasting. Marinate the haunch for twenty-four hours in red wine, bay leaves, rosemary, juniper and garlic; then slow roast until the meat is falling off the bone. Serve as a joint with braised red cabbage, dauphinoise potatoes and green beans. A large glass of claret, a roaring fire, and eyes will soon be glinting with wild desire.

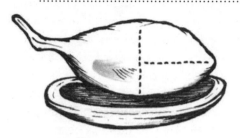

Slow Roast Haunch of Vension with Braised Red Cabbage

Venison haunch : small 1 kg joint
Juniper berries : 1 tbsp
Garlic : 4 cloves
Rosemary : 1 large sprig
Thyme : 1 small sprig
Bay leaves : 10
Red wine : ½ bottle
Butter . 100 g
Red cabbage : ½ head
Pears : 2
Vegetable oil . 1 tbsp
Redcurrant jelly : 1 tsp
Salt and pepper : to taste

Preheat the oven to 150°C.

Crush the juniper berries, smash the garlic and bruise the rosemary, thyme and bay leaves. Place in a large, lidded roasting pan with the joint of meat on top. Pour the wine over the top and cover. Refrigerate for 12 hours, turning occasionally.

Cut the butter into thin strips and place in the freezer to harden.

Remove the joint from the roasting pan, reserving the marinade. Pat dry and make deep incisions into the flesh with a sharp knife. Insert the frozen butter into the incisions.

Slice the red cabbage into 1 cm strips. Peel and core the pears and cut into 2 cm chunks. Mix the pear and red cabbage with the marinade.

Heat some oil in a large frying pan and sear the venison joint on all sides. Return to the roasting pan, making a hollow for it among the red cabbage. Cover the joint with a sheet of foil tucked closely against the meat. Cover the roasting pan with another sheet of foil tightly tucked into the edge, then place the lid on top.

Roast for 3 hours until very tender.

Unwrap the joint and keep warm. Pour off the liquid from the bottom of the pan. Remove the herbs from the red cabbage, crush the garlic and pear into a paste and mix through the braised cabbage. Season to taste with salt and pepper.

Skim any fat from the reserved roasting juice and strain into a saucepan. Place over a medium heat and boil until reduced by half to intensify the flavours. Mix through a teaspoon of redcurrant jelly to add sweetness to taste.

On a warm platter make a bed of the braised cabbage, place the rested venison haunch on top and serve with a gravy boat of sauce. The meat should be so tender that it falls off the bone.

Vegetables

ARTICHOKE

The vegetable in question is the globe artichoke rather than the knobbly, earth-dwelling Jerusalem variety. An important distinction to make as the Jerusalem artichoke is notable principally for an astounding ability to induce flatulence, potent enough to keep it firmly out of any aspiring Romeo's culinary repertoire. The globe artichoke is a different beast, praised as an aphrodisiac as far back as the misty time of the ancient Greeks.

The Greeks believed that Zeus transmogrified a former lover into the first artichoke plant. The legend tells of a randy Zeus spying a fair maiden innocently bathing on the shores of the Aegean island Zinari. Inflamed with passion, Zeus promptly ravished the young filly then and there. Cynara, as she was called, turned out to be seriously hot property; so much so that Zeus, besotted with his new playmate, made her into a goddess and installed her in Olympus, close at hand for extracurricular activity whenever his wife had her back turned. Despite its reputation as paradise, Cynara found that life in Olympus was not to her mortal tastes. Homesick, she soon began sneaking back to earth. When Zeus discovered this he assumed the worst. In a jealous rage he flung her out of Olympus and turned her into the spiky but lust-inducing plant we now know as the artichoke. From such sultry beginnings, the artichoke has been renowned for its arousing qualities from ancient times to modern America. In 1949 the Californian artichoke industry crowned a young Marilyn Monroe its first official Artichoke Queen. In sixteenth-century France artichokes were a pleasure reserved for gentlemen only. Their stimulating power was thought too potent for the wives and daughters of the day, who might become uncontrollable under the artichoke's saucy spell.

The artichoke plant is a member of the thistle family, the edible part being the flower bud. Integral to the plant's reproductive system, bulbous and full of pollen, it is easy to see why artichoke heads were first considered aphrodisiacs. Despite the vegetable's intuitive naughtiness, modern research has drawn something of a blank when trying to substantiate its historic claim to fame. Artichokes have been used extensively throughout history as a digestive aid, and to enhance liver function. Research into this phenomenon in the early twentieth century isolated a compound prevalent in artichokes, which is seriously handy if you have an unhappy liver: cynarin, named after Zeus's hapless squeeze, not only helps regenerate and protect the liver but also enhances overall liver function. This is all well and good and not terribly groundbreaking until you link it with more research indicating that a healthy liver is instrumental to maintaining a lusty sex drive.

One function of the liver is to regulate the manufacture of proteins. And one such protein is the wonderfully named globulin, which is needed to produce the hormone testosterone. Testosterone has a direct and decidedly enlivening effect on the libido, particularly in women. So it seems that our sixteenth-century French gents had good reason to restrict their women's artichoke intake. No self-respecting bourgeois *monsieur* wants sexual revolution. In fact, history's most legendary artichoke muncher, the famously man-eating Queen of France, Catherine de Medici, may have been such a virago precisely because her heroic consumption of artichokes induced an excess of testosterone.

Aside from their nutritional properties, artichokes make for some seriously sexy eating. Traditionally they are either steamed or boiled in a *court bouillon*, then served with melted butter, hollandaise or Béarnaise sauce. The leaves are plucked off one by one; each leaf base is then dipped in the sauce, popped in the mouth and the flesh scraped off with one's gnashers. Once the leaves are exhausted one needs some surgical skill to cut away the eponymous 'choke', which is the bristly unformed flower. Once this operation is complete, all that remains is to luxuriate in the most prized part of the artichoke, its delicious heart. This vegetable is far too sophisticated to give up its all on the first bite. First it coquettishly teases you with its leaves, giving up its pleasures morsel by morsel. Once stripped to its heart, resistance is over. Smear it with the remaining sauce and your mouth is rewarded with a sensory explosion of one of gastronomy's most unique and intense flavours.

....

Boiled Artichokes with Béarnaise Sauce

Large globe artichokes : 2
Lemon : 1
Bay leaves : 2
Black peppercorns : 4

Choose your artichokes carefully. They are generally best in summer. Select firm, heavy specimens with stiff, tightly furled leaves, which will vary in colour from green to violet depending on variety. Beware artichokes with black-tipped leaves; these not only look a bit sinister but, more practically, will have been picked some time previously. Remove the outer leaves of each artichoke, leaving the top two thirds in place. Break off the stalk, taking care to remove the stringy veins that come away with it – for this reason do not cut the stalk off with a knife. Wash under cold water and secure each artichoke's remaining leaves with a rubber band, so they will retain their shape while cooking.

Bring a large pan of water to the boil, add the juice of one lemon, the bay leaves and black peppercorns. Plunge your trussed artichokes into the water and boil vigorously for around 30 minutes.

The artichokes are ready when the remaining outer leaves come away with a firm downwards tug. Remove the rubber bands, drain for a few minutes in a colander and serve with warm béarnaise sauce.

BÉARNAISE SAUCE

Chopped chervil : 3 tbsp
Chopped tarragon : 3 tbsp
White wine vinegar : 75 ml
Chopped shallots : 20 g
Thyme : 1 small sprig
Bay leaf : 1
Black peppercorns : 3
Eggs : 2

Butter : 125 g
Lemon : 1
Salt and pepper : to taste

Place 2 tablespoons each of the chervil and tarragon in a small pan with the vinegar, shallots, thyme, bay leaf and peppercorns. Bring to the boil and reduce in volume by two thirds. Once the vinegar is reduced, strain out the herbs and spices.

Meanwhile crack your eggs, one-handed if possible (it's most impressive), and separate the yolks from the whites. Mix the yolks with 1 tablespoon of water and add to the reduced vinegar. Whisk together and heat very gently until the mixture thickens a little.

Melt the butter in a separate pan and gradually trickle the liquid butter into the eggs, whisking all the while. Go slowly, or the sauce will split and curdle.

Once all the butter has been added, the sauce should be the consistency of thick double cream. Add the remaining chervil and tarragon, a little salt and pepper if required and stir in a little lemon juice.

Serve the Béarnaise directly, or keep warm until needed – it cannot be reheated without splitting.

This sauce can be made less impressively, but more reliably, in a food processor. Simply mix the egg yolks in your food processor, add the strained vinegar reduction with the engine running, followed by a steady stream of melted butter, then the chopped herbs – almost too easy. To make a classic hollandaise, simply omit the tarragon and chervil.

ASPARAGUS

Asparagus, or 'grass' as my greengrocer insists on calling it, has long been considered to have magical lust-inducing properties. In the seventeenth century messianic English herbalist Nicholas Culpeper maintained that this tasty legume 'stirs up lust in man and woman', and looking at the evidence he may have had a point. Certainly asparagus's almost alchemical ability, in the words of Marcel Proust, to 'transform my chamber pot into a flask of perfume' indicates that this is not a vegetable to be trifled with.

The first spears thrust vigorously out of the earth in late April and continue thus until early June, thereby coinciding with nature's most fecund season. The birds and the bees have but one thing on their mind, and even we civilised sentients may feel a slight stirring of the loins. And asparagus itself does bear an uncanny likeness to a young man's primed pride and joy; ladies are said to prefer the fat white French variety rather than the slender green British version. I feel it my duty to point out to said ladies that although admittedly of inferior girth, the weedy British version has an infinitely superior taste, and is less prone to disease.

Not only tastier, the green asparagus wins hands down when it comes to nutrition, boasting an impressive arsenal of nutrients including vitamin A, potassium and folic acid. Potassium and vitamin A indirectly stimulate glandular and metabolic functioning, which in turn keeps one's sex drive firmly ticking over. Nice as this is, the true key to asparagus's lusty reputation may stem from its extremely high levels of folic acid. Folic acid triggers the body to produce histamines, an essential ingredient in reaching both the feminine oh-my-God moment, and the less-fair sex's grunting moment.

So far the evidence is pretty compelling: asparagus looks pretty lewd, has bolstering physiological effects and can be eaten only during nature's naughty season. And when it is eaten, asparagus is traditionally consumed in an undeniably louche manner. Forgoing prim cutlery, aficionados fingerly feed each other the warm slippery spears, which some debauchees further maintain one should gulp down whole without chewing like some sort of seasoned port professional.

To enjoy asparagus at its sensual best, stick to the British crop and get it as fresh as possible; there is nothing alluring about a wizened wilting spear. The best, freshest asparagus can be eaten raw, sliced with a mandolin into thin linguine-like strips. Serve as a salady side drizzled with truffle oil and sprinkled with sea salt. Otherwise, asparagus can be grilled, roasted, boiled or steamed. I prefer the latter two methods. They ensure that the spears remain plump and springy; but do be careful as they only take a few minutes and cannot bear overcooking.

Prepare the asparagus for the pot by washing thoroughly to remove any grit from the sandy soil in which they thrive. To be confident of grit-free asparagus, use a stiff bristled brush or knife to scrape off the outer membrane on the asparagus's skin, as this often harbours fine particles of dirt. Break off the woody stem by bending the spear up from the base until it snaps. Served simply with a knob of good-quality butter, asparagus is exquisite. This can be turned into something a little special using an anchovy and tarragon butter, or go the whole hog and make a beast of yourself serving your spears with a poached egg, bathed in hollandaise and topped with a ruffled slice of smoked salmon – probably better than the sex which will almost undoubtedly follow such a repast.

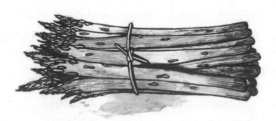

Asparagus with Poached Egg, Hollondaise and Smoked Salmon

The key to this dish lies in using the freshest asparagus and the freshest eggs. Asparagus behaves similarly to flowers or green herbs: once cut the stems will dehydrate rapidly, deteriorating in both flavour and appearance. They should be eaten no more than 72 hours from harvesting and should be stored in a refrigerator with a wet cloth wrapped around the cut ends. The freshness of one's egg is equally critical; when it comes to poaching, a fresh egg is essential. An old egg will have a loose runny albumen, which when placed in the poaching water may separate from the yolk, resulting in culinary catastrophe.

Hollandaise : 100 ml
Asparagus : 10 plump green spears
Chives : 5

White wine vinegar : 1 tbsp
Eggs (large) : 2
Smoked salmon : 2 slices
Sea salt : a pinch
Black pepper : to taste

Prepare your hollandaise sauce – follow the recipe for Béarnaise sauce on pages 84–5, omitting the tarragon and chervil. Keep warm for use later.

Wash your asparagus thoroughly and remove the woody stems; trim to a uniform length and tie into bundles of 5 spears. Finish your mise en place *by placing your plates in a warming oven and finely chopping the chives.*

Bring a large pan of salted water to the boil and place the bundles of asparagus upright in the pan. The tips should be just out of the water whilst the stems are fully submerged. Cover the pan and simmer gently for 4 or 5 minutes. The idea is that the stems boil while the more tender tips simultaneously steam. Slender spears will require a shorter cooking time.

Meanwhile in a wide shallow pan bring some water to the boil, add the vinegar and reduce the heat until scarcely simmering – so the surface of the water ripples gently but no bubbles form.

Note that eggs should be at room temperature, not used straight from the fridge. Crack an egg into a cup and gently slide the egg into the hot water. Cook for about 3 minutes for a runny yolk; if required one can gently fold the white over the yolk to create a neat, compact poached egg.

Once the egg is cooked to the desired degree, remove it from the water with a slotted spoon, refresh under cold running water, drain and trim off any excess white to leave a neat egg. Keep the finished egg warm in a pan of hot water, held at about 40°C, whilst you poach the second egg.

When the asparagus is cooked, drain well and shake off any excess water, untie each bundle and place in the middle of each warmed plate. Carefully place an artfully tousled slice of smoked salmon on the asparagus and put a poached egg on top of this.

Spoon warm hollandaise over the egg and garnish with a sprinkle of chives, a pinch of flaky sea salt and a grind of black pepper. Serve with a smile and some warm toasted English muffins.

....

AVOCADO

The avocado hails from Central America. For thousands of years the Mayans and Aztecs have loved out on its lusty properties. The very word avocado is laced with sexuality. It is derived from the Aztec word *ahuacatl* – which means testicle. Growing in pairs, two avocados dangling from a tree do bear a passing resemblance to a man's most sensitive section. In awe of the avocado's libidinous power, nubile princesses would scoff the buttery flesh in fertility rituals. During the harvest, protective fathers locked up their virgin daughters, fearful of avocado-induced impropriety.

Looking at it objectively, one must conclude that the Aztecs were on to something with the avocado. In addition to the powerful and convincing similarity-to-testes argument, there is something undoubtedly sensual about the curvaceous avocado with its velvety flesh, slippery stone and luxuriant flavour. Rather less suggestively, dietary research has uncovered a nutritional gold mine beneath the avocado's dark green skin. Avocados are awash with potassium and rich in vitamins E and B6. All three can help relieve stress and related sexual problems, specifically anxiety-induced infertility and impotence. Avocados will also help you look as sexy as they make you feel. High sterol levels in avocado oil boost collagen production, keeping skin soft, supple and springy, and lips of all description plump and pouting; all decidedly good things to those of conventional tastes.

Mashing avocados into guacamole, whilst tasty with tortilla chips, is not the best way to enhance their eroticism, particularly if you are male and share the Aztec belief in their testicular characteristics. I pant at the proposition of simply served avocado with buffalo mozzarella, ripe tomatoes and fresh basil, allowing one to luxuriate in their rich unctuousness. Should one's dining companion prefer their pleasure a little more primped, serve perfectly ripe avocado with fresh crab and samphire bound in a chervil mayonnaise and pressed into a chef's ring mould.

Avocado and Buffalo Mozzarella Salad
with Sweet Basil Dressing

The success of this dish relies on the ripeness of the avocado and on using good-quality mozzarella. Test the ripeness of your avocado by pressing firmly on to its skin with a finger – the flesh should give under this pressure. Another, and the ultimate, test, is to cut the avocado in half, remove the stone, and run a spoon inside the skin – one should be able to scoop out the entire flesh in one piece.

Fresh garlic : 1 small clove
Sea salt : 1 pinch
Palm (or brown) sugar : ½ tsp
White wine vinegar : 1 tbsp
Freshly squeezed lime juice : ½ lime
Extra virgin olive oil : 5 tbsp
Semi-dried tomatoes : 5
Chives : 1 tbsp
Sweet/Thai basil : 1 small bunch
Avocado : 1
Buffalo mozzarella : 1 (150 g)
Black pepper : to taste

Prepare the dressing by crushing the garlic with the salt and palm sugar into a fine paste in a pestle and mortar. Mix in a jar with the vinegar, lime juice and olive oil.

Finely slice the semi-dried tomatoes and the chives.

Chiffonade the basil: place the leaves on top of each other and roll up into a basil cigar, then finely slice to leave fine ribbons of bruise-free basil.

Add all three to the dressing jar, put a lid on and shake vigorously to combine.

Prepare the avocado and mozzarella salad, by first cutting the avocado in half. Remove the stone and using a spoon scoop out the flesh from each half in one piece. Slice the avocado lengthways into 5 mm slices.

Slice the mozzarella to the same thickness as the avocado and arrange on a serving plate, interleaving the avocado and mozzarella slices.

Pour the dressing over the avocado and mozzarella, grind some black pepper over the salad then cover with foil and leave the flavours to infuse for a couple of hours (while imbibing a well-deserved glass of Chablis). Serve with warm ciabatta and any remaining wine.

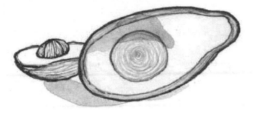

Avocado with Crab, Chervil and Samphire

Crab : 1 medium cooked crab

Semi-dried tomatoes : 6

Samphire : 100 g

Baby spinach : a large handful

Chopped chives : 1 tbsp

Chopped chervil : 1 tbsp

Mirin : 1 tsp

Tabasco : a few shakes

Mayonnaise : 5 tbsp

Lime juice : 2 tbsp

Avocado : 1

Sea salt : a pinch
Black pepper : a pinch
Cayenne pepper : a pinch

Either laboriously pick out the flesh from a freshly cooked crab or buy some ready-picked crabmeat from your fishmonger. If you are using your own crab, reserve the claws for decoration.

Finely chop the semi-dried tomatoes.

Blanch the samphire and baby spinach in boiling water for about 60 seconds. Refresh under cold running water and squeeze dry.

Finely chop the herbs. Reserve a little of the chopped herbs for garnishing and mix the rest with the crabmeat, samphire, spinach, tomato, mirin, Tabasco, mayonnaise and 1 tablespoon of the lime juice.

Select a ripe avocado, cut in half lengthways, remove the stone and using a large spoon scoop out the avocado flesh.

Slice the avocado thinly (3 mm) lengthways and brush with lime juice to stop the avocado discolouring from oxidisation whilst adding a zesty contrast to its butteriness.

Spread the sliced avocado across your plates. Place an oiled chef's ring next to the fanned avocado and press the crab mayonnaise into it. Remove the metal ring and top with a reserved cracked crab claw (if you have one).

Sprinkle some reserved chopped herbs, sea salt and freshly ground black pepper over the plate. Dust with a little ground cayenne pepper. Serve with a stack of hot buttered toast and start feeding each other.

BROAD BEANS

Until the discovery of the legume-rich New World, the broad bean was pretty much the only guest at an old-world bean feast. Cultivated since the Bronze Age, the broad bean went temporarily off the menu when ancient Greek mathlete Pythagoras theorised to his followers (of whom there were many) that beans were bad. Unlike his elegant mathematical theories, Pythagoras enigmatically gave no working whatsoever for his bean-banning conclusion.

The ancient world scratched its head and the ensuing debate brought out some of the biggest guns of the age: Aristotle, punching somewhat below his intellectual reputation, attributed the bean's forbidden status to its dubious similarity in shape to the male gonad; Cicero, Plutarch and St Jerome more astutely concurred that Pythagoras's animosity towards the broad bean was rooted in its supposed aphrodisiac properties, and the mathematician's prototypically prudish aversion to such matters. In addition to discovering remarkable properties about triangles, Pythagoras also founded a decidedly mysterious secret brotherhood of celibate, vegetarian mathematicians. The original secret society, this brotherhood has an unbroken history leading directly to the covert handshakes of today's Freemasons.

Chomped throughout Europe and Asia, broad beans enjoy a surely connected popularity in two of the world's most densely populated regions, northern China and the Egyptian Nile valley. They are the principal ingredient in the Egyptian national dish *fūl medames* and a key component in the ubiquitous felafel. Like most pulses, broad beans offer vegetarians a good source of protein and iron. Unlike other beans, they also contain the active amorous ingredient levodopa, a chemical the body uses to produce dopamine. As discussed previously, dopamine is the brain's reward and motivation hormone, dished out to drive us to fulfil our basic urges – the most base of which is to go and get frisky. So although not obviously sexy and unlikely to grace the table of lascivious lords, the humble broad bean has a lot to recommend itself to the lover, particularly to one on a budget. Fresh new-season broad beans steamed and served with mint, parsley, flaky sea salt and melted butter are a side dish that takes some beating; and for which a beating should be gladly accepted. Blitzed with lemon juice, olive oil, anchovy and Parmesan, broad beans make a delectable tapenade. Spread it on bruschetta, mix through pasta or serve dolloped on white fish.

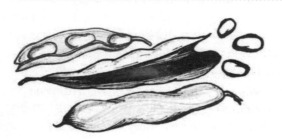

Broad Bean Tapenade

Broad beans require a bit of love to bring out their true glory. The bitter khaki foreskins need to be circumcised. Not the most engaging of culinary activities, so I would limit catering strictly to meals à deux.

Fresh broad beans (podded) : 250 g
Fresh garlic : 1 small clove
Sea salt : to taste
Salted anchovies : 4 fillets
Extra virgin olive oil : 50 ml
Lemon : ½ large lemon (unwaxed)
Chopped flatleaf parsley : 1 tbsp
Chopped mint : 1 tsp
Chopped basil : 1 tsp
Grated Parmesan : 1 tbsp
Black pepper : to taste

Steam the broad beans for 10 minutes. Refresh under cold water and set about removing the skins. I find the best way is to make an incision in the skin with a knife and gently squeeze out the beans.

Finely mash the garlic with the back of a knife and a little salt to make a smooth paste, add it to a small blender with the anchovies and a little olive oil. Pulse until they are combined.

Add half the beans, the juice of half a lemon and a teaspoon of finely grated zest to the garlic anchovy paste. Blitz until smooth.

Add the remaining ingredients and pulse to coarsely chop the beans and herbs into the tapenade.

Taste and season with freshly milled black pepper, sea salt and more lemon juice as required. If the tapenade is too stiff, mix through more olive oil.

CELERY

To the casual observer celery is a particularly joyless vegetable. Ninety-five per cent water, celery offers its dieting diners a positively misanthropic 6 calories per stalk. Hardly the ideal guest for a bon viveur's banquet, you would think. As it happens you would be wrong, for celery's other 5 per cent is pure rock and roll.

The jive is partly provided by some pretty active compounds called phtalides. Acting on the adrenal glands, they greatly reduce the production of stress hormones. Stress is one of the biggest causes of impotence, tightening blood vessels and strangling the libido. Phtalides have the net effect of loosening the tie, dilating the blood vessels and letting the love flow. They also directly increase testosterone levels. The adrenal glands produce 90 per cent of the body's DHEA, the chemical precursor to testosterone. When the adrenals are flat out producing stress hormones, DHEA production drops off. Conversely, when stress levels drop, DHEA and testosterone pick up.

If the phtalides provide celery's aphrodisiac rhythm, the keening front man is without doubt androstenone. This sex pheromone is nature's olfactory mating call. Broadcast at almost imperceptible levels from male armpits and groins, it touches a sensitive nerve in nubile nostrils, awakening the dark beast of female arousal. In an experiment, scientists secretly sprayed androstenone on to random seats in a theatre. Sending a gaggle of females into the theatre they observed where they sat. Unknowingly following their noses, our ladies nestled their behinds against the pheromone-scented seats. Celery is one of the few natural sources of androstenone. Putting away a few sticks of celery may increase a man's natural production of this love drug, making him quite literally irresistible to women. It may also explain why women are so fond of crudités and houmous.

Legend and history support the celery stick's aphrodisiac swagger. The blind bard Homer alludes to its pulling power in the *Odyssey*. Calypso the seductress nymph lived in celery-filled fields on the island of Ogygia. Rendered ravenous by her celery-heavy diet she pounced on the shipwrecked Odysseus, detaining him from his journey home for five years of fabled fornication. Central to the Celtic legend of Tristan and Isolde is a celery-filled love potion. By accident they drink this magic philtre and soon are rampantly rolling around, having completely forgotten that Tristan is escorting Isolde on her way to her wedding with his uncle.

Celery's use as a folk remedy for impotence had a particular following in France. In the eighteenth century Grimod de La Reynière, the world's first food journalist, warns of celery's aphrodisiac properties, advising that it 'is not in any way a salad for bachelors'. Madame de Pompadour, maverick mistress to Louis XV, fed celery soup to her monarch to raise the flagging royal standard. This practice continues today, in the potentially less elegant surroundings of the Ukraine. Brazen babushkas feed their pickled husbands hearty bowls of celery soup to ensure lusty performance.

Without wanting to upset any Ukrainian matrons, I would steer well clear of soup and recommend raw celery as most likely to cause maximum aphrodisiac effect. If we are talking raw celery our options are limited. Celery combines classically with apple and walnut in a Waldorf salad. A plump stick revels in the hot bath of a staunch Bloody Mary. Apart from that we can only really be contemplating crudités. I assume most people are au fait with how to prepare raw celery so I will set my culinary crosshairs on the ideal dip. Celery has an almost pregnant affinity for peanuts. Contrast the cool, wet crunch of the celery with the warming fire of a spicy satay sauce, so much more seductive than houmous.

Celery Crudités with Lime Satay Sauce

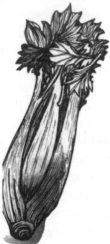

Celery : ½ head

Coriander : 10 g

Shallot : 1

Lime : ½

Dry-roasted peanuts (unsalted) : 90 g

Sunflower oil : 1 tbsp

Fish sauce : 1 tbsp

Tabasco : 1 tsp

Palm sugar / caster sugar : 10 g

Water : 75 ml

Dark soy sauce : 1 tsp

Toasted sesame oil : 1 tbsp

Remove the coriander leaves from the stalks and skin the shallot. Zest and juice the lime.

Crush the peanuts into small pieces using a rolling pin, then sauté the peanut pieces in a frying pan with the sunflower oil until golden brown.

Roughly chop the shallot and coriander stalks and place in a blender with the fish sauce, Tabasco, sugar, lime juice, lime zest, water, soy sauce and toasted sesame oil. Add three quarters of the peanuts and blitz until smooth.

Add the remaining peanuts and pulse to achieve a crunchy texture. If the sauce is too thick add a little water to loosen it.

Roughly chop the coriander leaves, stir into the sauce and chill to allow the flavours to develop. The sauce should be nutty and spicy with a delicious balance between sweet, sour and salt. You can adjust the seasoning to taste by adding more sugar for sweetness, more fish sauce for saltiness or lime juice for tartness.

Break the celery stalks away from the head, wash thoroughly and using a peeler cut off the strings that run along the ridges on the convex side of each stalk. Cut in batons about 10 cm long by 2 cm wide. Serve with the satay sauce for dipping.

FENNEL

Fennel is an under-appreciated ingredient. Like the pig, all its parts are deliciously edible. The seeds are a wonderful aromatic spice, the leaves an admirable herb, its fleshy bulb a versatile salad and vegetable side. Unlike the average curly-tailed snouter, fennel can drive women wild with desire.

It would appear that this particular characteristic was well known to the ancient Greeks. In *The Bacchae*, the illustrious playwright Euripides warns of 'brute wildness in the fennel-wands'. Fennel was closely associated with the disreputable Dionysus, god of wine and waywardness. Dionysus brandishes a phallic staff, or thyrsus; its shaft is a fennel stalk, its head a pine cone dripping with honey. His retinue is a rabble of wanton women and indecently aroused, prodigiously hung goat-men. At holy all-night raves, Dionysus's devotees wore crowns of fennel leaves, and chewed on fennel seeds to bring on the sacred desire.

Although this may well have worked for the wanton women, I suspect our engorged goat-men were on something else. Fennel's active ingredient is a phytoestrogen called anethole. It evolved as fennel's unorthodox defence against rampaging herbivores. Like a chemical kick in the balls, anethole zaps the male libido, ruining ruminant romance to keep the grazing population very much in check.

In humans, fennel's phytoestrogens have much the same effect. The literal translation of phytoestrogen, a Greek word, is a plant that creates sexual desire in women. These plant-generated oestrogens simply mimic the effect of animal sex hormones. In women, high oestrogen levels fuel a strong libido and womanly physique. In men it is a very different story. Normal oestrogen levels in males are very much lower. Increasing them sends men on a gender bender. Breasts swell, nipples enlarge, testicles shrivel and body hair falls out – interest in sex is an early casualty.

The gastronomic merits of fennel are many, but for the male bon viveur they come at a high price. Fennel is clearly an unsuitable staple for maintaining manliness. In Italy, as well as meaning fennel, *finocchio* is a somewhat derogatory term for a homosexual fellow. The term originated in the fifteenth century and is used to this day. The Renaissance Italian, none too politically correct, clearly had noted the un-manning effects in this otherwise admirable vegetable. I very much doubt, however, the odd salad and occasional slice of fennel salami will put breasts on your chest and take you to the wrong part of town. I indulge and am still a paragon of masculinity, albeit a somewhat flamboyant one who likes cooking. Run the gauntlet of a fennel's feminine charms and wow female companions with an exquisite fennel velouté served with a Parmesan and fennel-seed crisp.

....

Fennel Velouté with Fennel-Seed Parmesan Crisps

Fennel : 500 g

Onion : 1 small onion

Butter : 60 g

Bouquet garni : 1

Plain flour : 20 g

Chicken stock : 400 ml

Pastis : 1 tbsp

Star anise : 1

Egg : 1

Double cream : 3 tbsp

Salt : a pinch

Cayenne pepper : a pinch

Parmesan : 50 g

Fennel seeds : 2 large pinches

Whipping cream : 2 tbsp

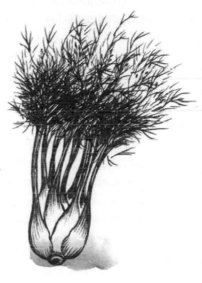

Preheat the oven to 180°C.

Finely slice the fennel and onion. Melt 20 g of butter in a pan and over a medium heat fry the vegetables with the bouquet garni for 10 minutes, stirring constantly.

Empty the pan and melt another 20 g of butter. Stir in the plain flour to make a white roux, then whisk in the chicken stock. Add the cooked vegetables, bouquet garni, pastis (Pernod is always a good one) and star anise. Bring to the boil and cook for 30 minutes at a light simmer.

Fish out the star anise and bouquet garni, then liquidise the soup in a blender until very smooth. If you want to be especially professional, now pass the soup back into the pan through a very fine sieve.

Crack and separate the egg, set the white aside and beat the yolk with the double cream.

Remove the soup from the heat and stir in the egg and cream. Finally whisk in the remaining 20 g of butter to give the soup a luxurious sheen.

Season with salt and a little cayenne pepper to taste.

To make the Parmesan crisps, grate the Parmesan. Sprinkle the cheese on to non-stick baking paper in two even circles, just wider in diameter than the bowls of the soup plates you are going to use.

Sprinkle the fennel seeds over each circle of Parmesan. Bake in the preheated oven for 5 minutes.

Once melted, remove from the oven, allow to cool then transfer to the freezer to set firm.

Serve the soup in warmed bowls with a swirl of whipping cream, dust with a little cayenne pepper and crown with the Parmesan crisp, which should hover over the soup like a lid.

TOMATO

Eighteenth-century France was a hotbed of decadence and debauchery. Bursting on to these licentious times, the scarlet tomato caused quite a splash. They were imported from Italy as *pommes d'amour* (love apples). The name, exoticism, sinful colour and juicy flesh were more than enough for them to be quickly accepted as powerful aphrodisiacs. Banished by the Catholic Church and unwelcome in polite society, they were embraced by everyone else.

Over the years, the aphrodisiac reputation faded and the love apple became the plain old tomato. Only in Italy does something of the original colourful name survive. The flamboyant Italians call tomatoes *pomodori*, or golden apples. The tomato's naughty French reputation turns out to have been a slip of the tongue. When the conquering Spanish returned from the New World, the Aztec *tomatl* that accompanied them were yellow not red. From Spain they spread to Italy and North Africa. Whereas in Italy the *pomodoro* remained yellow, in Moorish Africa a new red strain was developed. These were subsequently imported into Italy where they were known separately as *pomo dei mori*, apples of the Moors. When the French got their greedy mitts on them, this name was mistranslated into *pommes d'amour*, and so a slutty reputation was born.

Tomatoes remain rampantly red, they still ooze juicily from their meaty flesh, but only the most imaginative and hopeful still call them an aphrodisiac. Modern science may soon change that. A study at Harvard University has shown that men who eat tomatoes are a third less likely to contract prostate cancer.

The direct link to libido is as yet unclear. What is clear is that the prostate governs male sexuality and tomatoes make it tick. As an American scientist might say – you do the math. Make absolutely sure of aphrodisiac advantage with a Bloody Mary: tomato juice tooled up to the teeth with an X-rated arsenal of alcohol, chilli, pepper, anchovy essence, wasabi and celery. With that lot swilling around it is no wonder hungover sex is so splendidly satisfying.

Preparing the perfect Bloody Mary is an art everyone should master. It will be a friend for life. The bon viveur gives his stamp of approval to Little Devil, an ingenious Bloody Mary essence that packs all the punch of an expertly crafted cocktail but with a good deal less complication. Perfect for parlous mornings when it all seems a bit much, still better when you are in a rush to return to an occupied bed. If you have time on your hands, kick off an evening with a classy Bloody Mary variant, the incomparable Bloody Margarita, made with tequila, tomato liquor and lots of love.

....

Cheat's Bloody Mary

Vodka : 35 ml

Bloody Mary essence : 1 tbsp
(Little Devil pack in handy single servings)

Freshly squeezed lime juice : ¼ lime

Tomato juice : 200 ml

Celery : 1 stick

Pour the vodka, Bloody Mary essence, lime juice and chilled tomato juice into a glass. Trim the celery stick to an appropriate

*length, make a few lengthways incisions into one end, and use to
stir the cocktail together.*

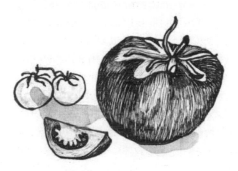

Bloody Margarita

Cherry tomato essence : 50 ml
(250 g cherry tomatoes and a stick of celery)

Silver tequila : 50 ml

Tabasco . ½ tsp

Fish sauce : ½ tsp

Amontillado sherry : 1 tbsp

Freshly squeezed lime juice : ½ lime

Celery salt : 2 tbsp

Black pepper : 1 tsp

Wasabi powder : 1 tsp

Salt : to taste

Ice : plenty

Cherry tomatoes : 2

*Make a tomato essence by pulsing 250 g of ripe cherry tomatoes
and a stick of celery in a food processor until they are very finely*

*chopped. Season with salt and pour into a sieve placed over a
bowl. Refrigerate for 3 hours, during which time a clear thin
liquid will have collected. Press the sieve to extract any remaining
essence.*

*Shake the tomato essence with ice, good-quality silver tequila,
Tabasco, fish sauce, sherry and lime juice.*

*Mix the celery salt with ground black pepper and wasabi
powder. Pour this on to a saucer, wet the rim of a cold Martini
glass and rub into the mixture.*

*Pour the margarita into the glass and serve with a cherry
tomato on a cocktail stick.*

....

TRUFFLES

In gastronomic circles the mysterious truffle inspires an almost
religious fervour. The illustrious French author Alexandre
Dumas described them as 'the holy of holies for the gourmet',
adding as an aside that they also 'make women more tender
and men more lovable'. D'Artagnan's creator was not the first to
notice this inimitable connection.

All the ancients were aficionados. Pyramid-potty Pharaoh
Cheops is said to have enjoyed truffles basted in goose fat. The
Babylonian kings preferred their truffles wrapped in papyrus
and cooked in ashes, like a ludicrously luxurious baked potato. The enlightened Greeks and Romans were more absorbed
by the truffle's aphrodisiac properties. From Pythagoras to
Plutarch, Marcus Aurelius to Aristotle, the great minds were
as one – truffles make you horny. This electric quality and

the truffle's inscrutable biology led to the belief that truffles were supernatural, appearing where lightning bolts struck the ground.

The Prophet Muhammad declared truffles to be a gift from Allah. Yet in Europe their consumption almost died out in the Middle Ages when the Church, bamboozled by obscure origins and ungodly groin goading, pronounced them evil. This embargo did not last long and with the Renaissance their popularity as gourmet guarantee of sexual satisfaction spread from royalty downwards. Soon the likes of Lucrezia Borgia, Catherine de Medici, Napoleon, Rasputin and the Marquis de Sade were all tucking in. Rehabilitation was complete when illustrious French gastronome Brillat-Savarin pronounced them 'the diamonds of the kitchen'; and when some of the mysteries of truffle cultivation were finally deciphered.

The truffle is the fruiting body of a microscopic fungal network that thrives among the roots of oak trees. Cultivation remains at best haphazard. Acorns gathered from truffle-bearing trees have a modest chance of growing into truffle trees themselves. The woolliness of the science is revealed when you learn that even today truffles are hunted as opposed to gathered; and that the truffle hunter is helpless without the keen nostrils of a four-legged friend.

Nothing tracks down a truffle like the sensitive snout of a randy sow. Truffles are catnip to pigs. They contain mega doses of porky sex pheromones, more than enough to bring Miss Piggy running, panting at the prospect of making bacon. The one drawback to truffling with pigs is that once the sexual mist descends it is hard to prevent your sizeable sidekick from gobbling the prize. Dogs can also be trained to sniff out truffles, but between you and me they lack the necessary motivation.

The truffle's complex earthy flavour and aroma engage and activate the senses in a way that is downright erotic. The aphrodisiac status is no doubt glossed by the truffle's lofty price tag. Money turns most people on and truffles cost a lot of wonga. Gambling tycoon Stanley Ho paid $330,000 for the world's largest truffle – a white monster weighing a hefty 1.5 kg. Dr Ho is perhaps living proof of the truffle's special powers. This Hong Kong-based octogenarian is a tango champion with four wives and seventeen children, the last of which he sired at the ripe old age of seventy-eight.

Those still doubtful can stick some science in their pipe and puff on that. It is not only pigs and truffles that produce the perfumed pick-me-up of androstenone. We also waft it from armpits and groins for much the same purpose. An experiment conducted by the University of Birmingham showed pictures of normally clad women to male and female subjects. Half of this group had been primed with a noseful of androstenone. The subjects were then asked to rank the women for sexual attractiveness. Those primed with pheromones gave significantly higher marks than the control group.

The black truffles of the Perigord have more androstenone than the white truffles of Alba and Istria. White truffles, however, are more expensive so the jury is out as to which offers the most aphrodisiac appeal. I have a mild preference for the subtler earthy tones of the Perigord truffle, rather conveniently at its best around Valentine's Day. Unleash its pulling power with a languorous linguine bathed in butter and spiked with an indecent amount of truffle. No point scrimping now, you may as well go the whole hog and wash it down with a classy red Burgundy of some pedigree and age.

....

Truffle Linguine with Savoy Cabbage and Lardons

Savoy cabbage . ½ head
Lardons/diced pancetta : 75 g
Butter : 50 g
Dry linguine : 200 g
Parmesan : 20 g
Egg : 1
Black Perigord truffle : 30 g
Salt and pepper : to taste

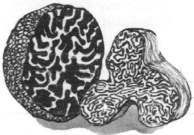

Remove any tough outer leaves from the savoy cabbage, then slice into thin linguine-like strips, lightly rinse and toss in a colander to dry.

Heat a lightly oiled frying pan and add the lardons. Cook for 5 minutes until the lardons are coloured and crisp.

Add the butter and once it has melted add the savoy cabbage. Toss in the butter for a minute then cover. Turn the heat down to low and cook for 8 minutes.

Meanwhile bring a large pan of salted water to the boil and cook the linguine for the required time.

Once cooked drain the pasta, and toss with the cabbage, lardons and grated Parmesan.

Crack and separate the egg, set the white aside and stir the yolk into the pasta. Season with salt and pepper as required.

Place a large pile of pasta on a plate and shave an indecent quantity of truffle on top.

Seafood

ANCHOVIES

The key ingredient in *pasta alla puttanesca* (prostitute's pasta), anchovies have long been considered a prelude to amorous activity. Anchovies themselves are a small marine fish that shoal in profusion across the globe's temperate seas, perhaps most notably in the western Mediterranean. Although eaten fresh and marinated in vinegar as *boquerones*, anchovies are principally preserved in oil following a gutting, salting and maturing process. The preserved anchovy fillet is not for the faint-hearted palate, packing a gutsy, salty, savoury flavour and a nostril-engulfing fishy fragrance. The intense taste and aroma could certainly be considered sexy in a visceral, down-and-dirty kind of way; not exactly nice, but nasty is surprisingly popular.

The most notable nutritional feature of anchovies is their high level of the B-complex vitamin niacin. Sexual function is predominantly controlled by the endocrine system of glands, principal of which is the pituitary gland. These glands secrete the hormones that flowing around our bodies get us hot and bothered, firm and frisky and generally unable to concentrate on the matter in hand, unless of course one's matter is already in one's hand. In order to function properly and produce sufficient hormones these glands have specific nutritional needs. The pituitary gland requires supplies of zinc, vitamin E, and last but not least B-complex vitamins, including niacin. A deficiency in the pituitary causes underdeveloped sex organs, early menopause in women and impotence in men, three various but equally alarming outcomes. Niacin has in addition a specific importance as it cannot be stored by the body for future use, so must be frequently replenished through regular consumption of, amongst other things, *pasta alla puttanesca.*

This dish has its origins in the bordellos and bawdy houses of Naples. It is a spunky tomato-based sauce flavoured with anchovies, chilli and garlic, then mixed through with chopped capers, black olives and basil. The anchovies are not solely responsible for this sauce's X-rated reputation; garlic, chilli and basil are all aphrodisiacs in their own right. There are various explanations as to the dish's naughty name; its hot spicy flavour and pungent smell is certainly redolent of exotic ladies of the night and their not-so-fresh fragrance. Some say that whereas your average Italian mamma would shop daily for fresh produce, your average Neapolitan whore was kept hard at it, and so had to rely on long-life store-cupboard staples for her daily meals. People who believe this are perhaps a little dull. I prefer to believe that the dish brings out one's inner harlot, the one lurking secretly in every starched white shirt and prim and proper bodice.

....

Pasta alla Puttanesca
Ripe plum tomatoes : 400 g (or one can of tinned tomatoes)
Fresh red chilli (mild) : 1
Garlic : 3 fat cloves
Sea salt : to taste
Extra virgin olive oil : 100 ml
Salted anchovy fillets : 6
Capers : 2 tbsp

Black olives : 12
Basil : a small bunch
Dried penne pasta : 250 g

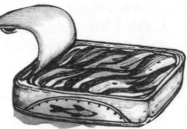

Roughly chop the tomatoes,
finely slice the red chilli and mash
the garlic clove into a paste with
a little sea salt.

Heat the olive oil and add the garlic, chilli and anchovies. Fry
for 2 minutes, then add the chopped tomatoes. Bring the sauce
gently to the boil.

Meanwhile rinse the capers and roughly chop with the pitted
black olives.

Once the sauce is simmering add the chopped capers and
olives and let the sauce gently reduce for 20 minutes.

Chiffonade the basil: place the leaves on top of each other
and roll up into a basil cigar, then finely slice to leave fine
ribbons of bruise-free basil.

Boil the pasta (traditionally spaghetti, but for me the sauce
clings better to penne) with a little oil in plenty of salted water,
for the prescribed time. Then drain.

Add the pasta to the tomato sauce. Stir to combine – then
serve sprinkled with the ribbons of fresh basil.

CAVIAR

Ethically dubious, cripplingly pricey and irresistibly alluring, caviar is the black ace in the aphrodisiac pack. The very word caviar hints at extraordinary properties, derived from the Persian word *kawyar* or cake of strength. History is littered with tsars, shahs, kings and emperors who have slurped from this fishy font. The roll call includes such lecherous luminaries as Casanova and Rasputin who would prime themselves for nights of passion with gobs of this esoteric delicacy. Frank Sinatra liked to keep the party going into the morning. He would prep Ava Gardner for a louche lie-in with the most decadent of breakfasts: caviar and scrambled eggs.

Caviar is the salted unfertilised eggs of the stately sturgeon. Prehistoric in origin, the most prized Beluga sturgeon can grow to a massive 5 metres in length and a groaning 2 tonnes in weight. Although sturgeon feed in the nutrient-rich waters near river deltas and estuaries, they head into fresh water to spawn. Fishermen lie in wait to ambush the females. A hefty whack to the fishy forehead stuns the mum-to-be whilst the flick of a rusty blade cuts out the ovaries in the crudest of oophorectomies. The black bounty of briny eggs can weigh up to 10 per cent of the fish's total body weight. The eggs are washed, sieved, lightly salted and finally packed into those tiny lithographed tins, which are so bewilderingly expensive.

Until recently, tucking into a can of caviar came with an uncomfortable burp of ethical indigestion. The unfortunate sturgeon seldom survives the brutish egg extraction. To make matters worse, sturgeon spawn only every five years, and only when they reach twenty years old. The most expensive caviar comes from the largest and most ancient fish. Unsurprisingly, unscrupulous over-fishing has pushed stocks of wild Caspian sturgeon to the point of extinction. Fortunately, international fish farming has saved us all from caviar catastrophy. Caviar is now humanely harvested from a variety of sturgeon strains comparable in quality to the wild Beluga, Ossetra and Sevruga of the Caspian Sea. Farming has also brought the price of caviar down. The most prized white Almas Beluga is packed in a 24-carat gold tin and can cost an oligarchic $25,000 per kilogram. By comparison Prunier's French farmed caviar is almost egalitarian, costing 'just' $1,700 per kilogram.

As any hedge fund manager will attest, wealth is an aphrodisiac. As one of the most expensive delicacies available, it is no surprise that caviar has quite the reputation too. The allure of the stinking rich is amplified by a wonderful set of rituals to enhance and announce one's conspicuous consumption. Serve in a cut crystal bowl placed on a bed of ice with a softly gleaming mother-of-pearl spoon jutting from your black hoard. Connoisseurs, such as myself, insist that caviar should be eaten off human skin. Make a loose fist, place a small spoonful of caviar on the soft skin between your forefinger and thumb, and revel in the seamy suggestiveness as your inamorata slurps it up. Once in the gob, caviar's true charms are revealed. Caviar may be expensive but then again it is undeniably delicious, offering a uniquely sensuous eating experience. The sensation is silky smooth and unctuous with a delicate savoury marine flavour. Pop the tiny eggs with your tongue and you are rewarded with bursts of creamy nutty nuance.

The sensuality of caviar and its high status are aided and abetted in the aphrodisiac stakes by an incredible array of nutritional goodies. It is a good source of calcium and phosphorus, as well as protein, selenium, iron, magnesium, and vitamins B12, B6, B2, B44, C, A and D. All excellent but it is the payload of amino acids arginine and histidine that provide the bang for your buck. Arginine acts in a very similar way to Viagra, speeding the rush of lewd blood into rude regions – stiffening male resolve and intensifying ecstatic exclamations. Histidine is required for triggering and lengthening orgasms in both men and women, and is directly responsible for the sexual flush that spreads across chests in exquisite moments of extremis.

When it comes to serving caviar it is best to focus one's culinary creativity on the supporting cast rather than the star turn. It is hard to improve upon perfection. The traditional accompaniment is blinis – small Russian buckwheat pancakes. Never afraid to fly in the face of received opinion, I prefer to partner my caviar with perfectly petite potato pancakes. Serve your pancakes with sour cream, and alternate morsels of the black stuff with nibbles of this tasty counterpoint and sips of bone-dry champagne.

Potato Blinis

Floury potatoes : 150 g
Onion : 1 small sweet bulb
Butter : a good knob
Milk : 75 ml
Egg (large) : 1
Self-raising flour : 40 g
Salt : ½ tsp
Sugar : ½ tsp
Vegetable oil : 1 tbsp

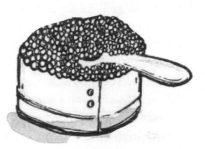

Peel the potatoes and cook in salted, simmering water until soft. Drain and mash until very smooth.

Meanwhile slice the onion very finely, and gently sweat it in a pan with a little butter until cooked through.

Whisk the mashed potato with the milk, onion and the yolk of the egg. Once these are combined add the flour, salt and sugar and whisk together.

Whisk the egg white until it is stiff. Fold half the egg white into the batter using a metal spoon, then carefully fold in the remainder, trying to keep the batter as fluffy as possible.

Heat a little oil in a frying pan and place small spoonfuls of batter into the pan. Cook the pancakes over a medium heat for about 3 minutes on each side until golden brown. The ideal pancake should be about 4 cm in diameter and about ½ cm thick.

THE SONG OF THE VIRGIN STURGEON — ANON

Caviar comes from the virgin sturgeon
A virgin sturgeon is a very fine fish
Virgin sturgeon needs no urgin'
That's why caviar is my dish.
I fed caviar to Louisa
She's my honey tried and true
Now Louisa needs no urgin'
I recommend caviar to you.
I fed caviar to my grandpa
He was a man of ninety-three;
Screams and cries were heard from grandma,
Grandpa had her up a tree.
I fed caviar to my sweetheart,
She always did it cheerfully.
Now she does it with a vengeance,
Oh, my God, it's killing me.
I put caviar in the punchbowl,
That livened up the party, sure.
What am I doing stripped down naked?
Thought these girls were sweet and pure.

LOBSTER

Aphrodisiacs are named after Aphrodite, the splendidly sexual Greek goddess of love. She was born of the sea, appearing from the deep fully formed and gloriously naked on a splayed scallop shell. Since antiquity, all shellfish has been associated with Aphrodite, rightly regarded as food for love. Lobster is the daddy of the shellfish family and has a suitably heavyweight aphrodisiac reputation. It is the most luxurious and expensive crustacean, a lavish indulgence to melt the heart with a spot of spoiling. Add a romantic red shell, an indecently suggestive aroma, and a viscerally sensual, hands-on eating experience – lobster is hot to trot. It is the Scarlett O'Hara of *fruits de mer*. Last but by no means least, lobster also tastes absolutely delicious.

Although lobsters are found all over the world, it is the cold seas of the North Atlantic that house the most delicious, big-clawed varieties. The European or common lobster is found mainly on the rocky coastline of France, Britain and Norway. The larger northern lobster flourishes most famously in Maine on the eastern seaboard of the USA. These kings of the sea have blue blood and can live almost indefinitely. Perhaps hinting at their aphrodisiac potential, as lobsters get older they become increasingly fertile. The largest lobster ever caught was a 20-kg monster. At his age he must have been quite the old goat.

Lobsters may be randy but they are also surprisingly romantic. It is the female lobster who picks her beau. The male ushers her into his rocky hole, where she then performs a protracted striptease, taking up to an hour to slip out of her shell. Once she is naked the magic happens. Rather touchingly, the gallant gentleman lobster will then guard his lover for a few days while her new shell hardens. Possibly flush with love, the sweetest-tasting lobsters are females who have just shed their shell. Hard-shell lobsters, although the easiest to transport and the most commonly eaten, are also the toughest. Lobsters grow by shedding their shell. Their flesh becomes denser and denser until, too tight, the lobster is forced out of its shell. Once naked, the lobster softens and expands by absorbing water. A new soft shell forms, hardening gradually over the following year.

The lobster is conspicuously absent from gastronomic history, largely because until the invention of the lobster pot in 1808 they were damn hard to catch. The only other method is diving, and it seems not many people fancied a lung-busting plunge in the freezing waters of the North Atlantic. In Europe, they were a luxury reserved for royalty and aristocrats. In America, they didn't really know what to do with the bounty from their newly invented lobster pots. Lobster was food for fish hooks and fertiliser, not fine living. Servants in Maine would insist in their employment contracts that they were not to be fed lobster more than twice a week. The late-nineteenth-century fad for seaside summer vacations, and fancy folk from Boston and New York, are what put lobster on America's gastronomic map. These cosmopolitans propagated the reputation of Maine lobster. Soon surf 'n' turf and lobster Thermidor were feeding the finest in the land. Rapacious over-fishing was all it took for the once-plentiful lobster to ascend to its current position as one of the world's most luxurious foods.

Like scallops, crab and langoustine, lobsters boast all the

goodness of the sea. They are stocked with a particularly nutritious larder of libido-enhancing minerals, vitamins and amino acids. Zinc is essential to sexual satisfaction and lobsters have got loads of it (see oysters for more detail). Selenium is also a bonus. This mineral is vital to male fertility. Concentrated in the testicles it breeds the strongest of little spermy swimmers. The rich array of B vitamins is equally beneficial to healthy production of the various sex hormones. Lobster has a full set of amino acids, including a boatload of arginine. Used as a chemical treatment for impotence, arginine stimulates the production of nitric oxide, transforming limp lengths of useless gristle into towering beacons of masterful masculinity. Left-out lady readers will be pleased to hear that arginine's effects are very much equal opportunity.

A lobster dinner should be a spectacle. Wrestling your dinner, winkling out titbits and licking your fingers are all part of the fun. Lobster is typically boiled or grilled. I find the drama, flavour and frivolity are all enhanced by roasting your lobster in a carefully constructed carapace of greaseproof paper, filled with herbs, spices, vegetables and a splash of white wine. Bring the lobster to the table in its bag, cutting into the paper to release a sensuous sauna of lobster-scented steam. Alternatively, allow the lobster to cool in its bag, perform the necessary culinary surgery and serve formally on a platter with roast garlic mayonnaise, a green salad and warm potato salad.

No morsel of a delicacy like lobster should go to waste. Use the shell, tomalley (the soft, green flesh in the body cavity) and roasting detritus to create a luxurious lobster bisque fortified with a splash of cognac. Perfect from a Thermos for a romantic spring picnic on a blustery day by the sea. It is as Aphrodite would have wanted.

....

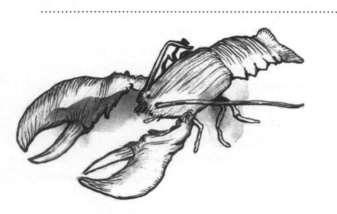

Lobster in a Bag

If you are cooking lobster yourself you need to buy it alive and perform the last rites in-house. The most humane way to snuff out the crustacean's flickering flame is to slowly freeze it to death. Wrap the lobster in a plastic bag and place in the deep freeze for 2 hours. Plunge the icy lobster's head into rapidly boiling water for 60 seconds to make sure of the execution.

Lobster : 1 large lobster (or two small 500g lobsters)
Garlic : 2 cloves
Carrots : 2
Celery : 2 sticks
Fennel : 1 head
Onion : 1 medium onion

Thyme : 1 sprig
Parsley : 1 small bunch
Bay leaf : 1
Cloves : 2
Star anise : 1
Cayenne pepper : a pinch
Butter : 50 g
Dry white wine : a large glass
Salt and pepper : to taste
Greaseproof paper

Preheat the oven to 230°C.

Crush the garlic and finely slice the carrots, celery, fennel and onion. Mix with the herbs and spices and place on two sheets of greaseproof paper.

Melt the butter, and use to brush the recently deceased lobster. Place the lobster on the bed of vegetables, season and pour the white wine around it. Wrap the greaseproof paper around the lobster and vegetables to create a loose but firmly secured airtight parcel – if necessary fasten with string.

Bake the lobster in the preheated oven for 45 minutes – if you are cooking two smaller lobsters 30 to 35 minutes should be sufficient. The roasted vegetables can be reserved for the Lobster Bisque recipe (see page 128).

Prepare the cooked lobster (at the table if you are serving it hot) by splitting it lengthways with a knife. Remove the digestive tract that runs down the length of the tail, crack the claws and get stuck in. It is generally advisable to give the head and body cavity a miss. The greenish tomalley, which is the liver and pancreas, is often held up to be the most aphrodisiac part of the lobster but it is also a bit grisly-looking and intense for some.

Classic Lobster Bisque

Lobster carcass : 1
Butter : 25 g
Brandy : 4 tbsp
Risotto rice : 50 g
Cooked vegetables : see recipe for Lobster in a Bag
Water : 1 litre
Tomato puree : 2 tbsp
Crème fraîche : 100 ml
Cayenne pepper : to taste
Salt and pepper : to taste

Remove the tomalley from the lobster carcass, then in a bowl pound the shells with the end of a rolling pin until well crushed.

Melt the butter in a wide shallow pan then add the lobster shell. Fry for 30 seconds, then add the brandy and flambé.

Add the rice together with the vegetables, herbs and spices reserved from the lobster in a bag recipe. Stir to combine, then pour over the water and mix in the tomato puree. Bring to the boil, then simmer for 35 minutes.

Strain the bisque through a fine sieve, pressing as much vegetable paste through the sieve as possible. Return to the pan and boil vigorously to reduce the bisque to about 500 ml of liquid.

Whisk in the reserved lobster tomalley and crème fraîche. Season with cayenne pepper, salt and pepper as required.

MUSSELS

Mussels are the poor man's oyster. Much beloved by our Belgian brethren, these briny little bivalves lack celebrity but offer the same aphrodisiac array of nutrients as their better-known big brother. The same bang for considerably less buck – cheap-date, bon viveurs take note. The inexpensive mussel holds its head up high, fine enough to bring a blush to the most high-falutin' dining companion. Those that shudder at the raw kiss of a freshly shucked oyster will also appreciate the down-to-earth, conventional charms of the cooked mussel. Share a steaming cauldron of mussels with a loved one and the sensual pleasure of slurping tender morsels from hard shells will budge the most barnacled of libidos.

Mussels grow in clusters at the low tide line of rocky shores. Although they have been a food source for thousands of years, the history of mussel cultivation begins in thirteenth-century France. In 1290 a shipwrecked Irishman, Patrick Walton, was washed up on the French coast near La Rochelle. His enquiring Celtic mind noticed that the posts set up in the shallows to catch seabirds were covered with mussels. He planted posts close together, slung branches (*bousches*) between them and watched with satisfaction as his invention yielded bumper crops of mussels. The *bouchot* method of mussel cultivation carries on to this day.

As with oysters (and cockles and clams), mussels derive their aphrodisiac goodness from lusty marine minerals and two rather special amino acids. In the run-up to spawning, aspartic acid and methyl-aspartate pump mussels full of fertility.

Following the throw-enough-mud-and-some-of-it-will-stick philosophy, mussels procreate by belching out superhuman quantities of sperm and eggs. In the vast sexual soup of speed-dating they hope at least some relationships will form before the whole lot gets washed out to sea. Studying baskets of fresh bivalves from the fish markets of Naples, scientists from Barry University in Miami and the Naples Institute of Neurobiology identified these two rare amino acids. They injected rats with them and observed supercharged rodent libido and raised levels of both testosterone and progesterone. The mineral X-factors are zinc, folic acid and selenium. They all are equally necessary to tip-top titillation and in-depth satisfaction (see oysters, asparagus and lobster for more detail).

When it comes to rustling up a cut-price aphrodisiac dinner, *moules marinières* is a hard dish to beat. Easy, effective and un-taxing on the wallet, it is the definition of a one-pot wonder. Mussels, parsley, white wine and cream, twenty minutes of cooking and you are ready to roll. In Britain, the white wine is traditionally substituted with cider to equally delicious effect. My version dispenses with both, balancing the mussels' sweet salty flavour with a mild, creamy curry sauce flavoured with saffron, ginger, curry leaf and coriander. Serve in a commu-nal bowl with crusty bread to soak up the sauce and a young Muscadet to wash it down.

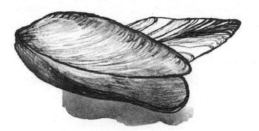

Saffron and Coconut *Moules Marinières*

Fresh coriander : 1 small bunch
Garlic : 2 cloves
Ginger root : 2 cm length
Carrot : 1 small carrot
Onion : 1 small onion
Mussels : 1 kg
Mustard seeds : a large pinch
Coriander seeds : a large pinch
Cumin seeds : a large pinch
Butter : 50 g
Curry leaf : a large pinch of dried leaves or 3 fresh leaves
Saffron : 8 strands
Coconut milk : 150 ml
Double cream : 100 ml

Roughly chop the coriander stalks and root, crush the garlic, and finely slice the ginger, carrot and onion. Wash the mussels under cold running water, pulling the beards off and discarding any that remain open.

Heat the spice seeds in a dry pan, then grind to powder in a pestle and mortar.

Melt the butter in a large pan, then sauté the vegetables with the ground spices, curry leaf and coriander stalk.

Hydrate the saffron in 50 ml of boiling water and leave to infuse for a few minutes.

Once the onion is soft add the coconut milk and saffron water, then bring to the boil. Put the mussels in the pan, cover and steam for 5 minutes.

Remove the mussels from the pan and discard any unopened specimens.

Strain the sauce through a fine sieve, return to the pan, mix in the cream and the reserved coriander leaf. Return the mussels to the pan and toss in the sauce.

Serve immediately.

....

OYSTERS

Oysters are aphrodisiac superstars. Everyone and their dog knows there is something special about these briny sex-bombs. I have slurped my way through more than my fair share, and am loudly confident that the fire fuelling this smoky reputation is red hot.

In many ways oysters are unlikely aphrodisiacs. They belong to the same biological family as slugs, feed off plankton and live in the brackish shallows of somewhat desolate estuaries. Unlike slugs, oysters are awe-inspiringly fertile. They may only come once a year but when they do it is an atomic sexual explosion.

A single oyster can produce over a million eggs and enough sperm to turn the sea milky white. They are so supercharged they can even fertilise themselves!

Man has availed himself of this coastal superfood since pre-historic times. Huge piles of discarded shells show that Cro-Magnon man was quite the bon viveur. The Romans were the first to truly wallow in the oyster's erotic delights. Ladies would dip oysters in honey as an incendiary hors d'oeuvre to lustful nights of imperial decadence. Emperor Vitellus was a consummate connoisseur, shipping snow-covered baskets of the finest British oysters to feed his refined appetite. Fast forward to the Enlightenment and we find oysters' aphrodisiac allure undiminished. Legendary Venetian lothario Casanova would fuel himself for a busy day at the orifice with the original breakfast of champions, five dozen of our friendly bivalves.

The oyster's scandalous reputation has both psychological and nutritional foundation. Eating a raw oyster enrages the senses with steamy stimuli. The smell, taste and texture allude to carnal matters – oceanic, wet, squelchy, soft and silky smooth. Put simply, if anything is sex on a plate, oysters are it. Lean, mean and full of beans, they harbour a sizzling low-fat cocktail of zinc, iodine and amino acids. A nutritional mix that specifically nourishes the two main drivers of desire: rapacious manly testosterone and orgasm-craving dopamine.

As oysters limber up for the heroics of the mating season, like mussels they flood with two rare amino acids, aspartic and methyl-aspartate. In humans, these acids perform much the same job, raising testosterone levels and stiffening sexual resolve. The massive zinc levels in oysters amplify this effect, arresting testosterone's natural synthesis into wimpy, pyjama-clad oestrogen. The dopamine effect is equally strong, boosted by oysters' richness in another amino acid called tyrosine. This metabolises directly into dopamine. High dopamine levels trigger an irresistible impulse and reward circuit in the primal brain, goading otherwise civilised citizens to rut in cupboards like beasts.

Oysters offer more than just sexual inspiration and enjoyment. In their extraordinary zinc content they provide the ejaculatory arsenal to arm the most protracted bedroom battle. When a man (or indeed a woman) huffs and puffs and gasps then gushes, that gush will contain 1–3 mg of zinc. If you want to gush again any time soon, either ensure you have stockpiled enough zinc to draw on reserves or reload at your nearest oyster bar.

Oysters are at their aphrodisiac best in the spring run-up to the spawning season. To bask in their gourmet and nutritional goodness, you cannot be squeamish. Oysters must be eaten raw and they must be alive. They have no central nervous system so this is not as heartless as it may initially seem. Aliveness is imperative. The deceased oyster decays at a rapid rate, and a night of the runs is rarely romantic. Oysters should be bought as fresh as possible and eaten immediately. Store on ice in the fridge with a wet tea towel covering your haul. Test each oyster before you open it. The shell should be tightly closed and heavy with water. Some dead oysters may also be closed but can be identified by the distinctive hollow clacking sound they make when tapped.

The classic way to serve oysters is freshly shucked on the

half-shell, chilled on a bed of ice and accompanied by bread and butter. The complex ozone, mineral taste and creamy, yielding flesh is usually tempered by a condiment of some sort. The most commonly served are lemon juice, black pepper, Tabasco and shallot vinegar. I have used elements of them all in the creation and refinement of my own inestimable Sauce Bon Viveur. When I need a break from blowing my own trumpet, I look east for inspiration and wolf down a delightful dozen with a zingy watermelon and daikon salsa.

SHUCKING OYSTERS

Opening an oyster is not the easiest of tasks. Place the oyster curved side down on a bunched-up dishcloth. Holding the oyster securely, firmly wiggle the blade of a stout oyster knife into the hinge joining the two halves of the shell. Once the point is securely lodged, twist the blade until there is a slight pop as the top shell is prised open. Slide the knife across the top shell to cut the adductor muscle. The lid can now be removed and the oyster loosened from the bottom half of its shell ready to be slipped effortlessly between one's salivating lips. To avoid getting any unexpected titbits of shell, you can strain the juice from the oysters into a bowl. Remove the oysters from the shell and wash both under cold running water. Replace the oysters in the shells and spoon a little reserved juice over each one.

Sauce Bon Viveur

Spring onion : 2
Mild red chilli : 1
Butter : 15 g
White wine vinegar (good quality) : 50 ml
Dry white wine : 50 ml
Honey : 1 tsp
Freshly squeezed lemon juice : 1 tbsp
Tomato puree : 1 tbsp

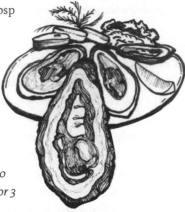

Wash two large spring onions, deseed the red chilli and slice both as finely as possible.

In a small saucepan heat the butter until it melts and starts to foam.

Add the spring onion and chilli to the foaming butter and fry gently for 3 minutes.

Add all the remaining ingredients, remove from the heat and whisk together.

(NB Make sure you use a good-quality white wine vinegar in this recipe.)

Set the sauce aside to cool thoroughly to allow the flavours to develop, then pass through a fine sieve to leave a silky-smooth sauce.

Chill and serve about half a teaspoonful with each freshly shucked oyster.

Watermelon and Daikon Salsa

Carrot : 1 tbsp diced carrot
Cucumber : 1 tbsp diced cucumber (see below)
Watermelon : 1 tbsp diced watermelon
Daikon : 1 tbsp diced daikon (see below)
Ginger root : 1 tsp finely chopped
Fresh coriander : 1 tsp finely chopped
Mirin : 75 ml
Rice vinegar : 50 ml
Honey : to taste (½ tsp)

Like many things Japanese, this recipe is pretty as a picture but calls for slightly obsessive precision. The vegetables need to be very finely and very neatly diced.

Peel and de-seed the cucumber before dicing, and use only a firm piece of watermelon.

Daikon is a large parsnip-shaped Japanese radish also known as mooli. This needs to be peeled and diced as before. If you can't lay your hands on daikon, a European pink radish will suffice.

The ginger and leaf coriander need to be chopped as finely as possible.

All that remains is to mix the ingredients together and sweeten to taste with honey.

Chill and serve as before, about half a teaspoonful per oyster.

PUFFERFISH

After the golden poison frog, the pufferfish is the most toxic creature on earth. Each fish contains enough poison to kill thirty men and there is no known antidote. Undeterred by these dubious accolades, the Japanese have prized pufferfish or fugu as an aphrodisiac delicacy for thousands of years. It is clear that the kamikaze spirit is very much alive and well.

The poison in pufferfish is a substance called tetrodotoxin, roughly ten times more venomous than cyanide. Tetrodotoxin poisoning results in numbness followed by paralysis. As the poison cannot cross the blood–brain barrier the stricken gourmet will savour eventual suffocation fully conscious. Dicing with death lies at the heart of pufferfish's aphrodisiac reputation. In small doses tetrodotoxin causes a pleasurable light-headedness, numb lips and a delightful tingling to fingers, toes and certain other manly extremities. Said manly extremities are also strengthened with the righteous rigidity of partial paralysis.

The trick with preparing pufferfish is to remove the poisonous organs whilst leaving just enough tetrodotoxin to foster some risky romance. This is no task for the amateur. The poison is distributed across the fish's skin, intestines, eyes, kidneys, ovaries and, above all, in its liver. Fugu's preparation is strictly controlled. Sushi masters must successfully complete three years of special training before they can prepare fugu for the public. People still die from fugu poisoning but most fatalities are the result of enthusiastic amateurs coming a cropper when indulging in culinary DIY.

The element of danger no doubt adds to the pufferfish's aphrodisiac allure. The boost of adrenaline will stoke the pit of desire as efficiently as the hopefully mild poisoning. Typically fugu is served as sashimi, cut into wafer-thin translucent slices that are artfully arranged as chrysanthemum flowers. The taste is extremely mild with a hint of chicken. Taste, however, is almost incidental to the experience. Dining on pufferfish is a spectacle. The chef will ceremoniously dissect a living pufferfish, pulsing in pieces, in front of your eyes. The flesh is used for sashimi whilst its fishy balls – the most aphrodisiac part of the whole creature – are served in hot sake. It is illegal to serve the toxic liver. Nevertheless, if pressed, a chef will often oblige with an under-the-counter sliver of gourmet death wish. The tingling is palpable, distinctly dangerous and overwhelmingly seductive.

Pufferfish is the only food denied to the Japanese Emperor and his family. Unless you are in a licensed restaurant I suggest you follow his imperial lead. If you are in the right surroundings, roll the dice and relish in the aphrodisiac tingle of knowing that just maybe this might be your last meal. There is no better way to feel triumphantly alive.

SEA URCHIN

The spiny sea hedgehog is a gourmet gift to intrepid lovers, and one of my absolute favourites. The rich iodine intensity of sea urchin roe is a unique flavour that invigorates immediately. More than any other nation, the Japanese share my enthusiasm. In the Land of the Rising Sun sea urchins, or uni, have been treasured as an aphrodisiac for thousands of years. Sadly, the rocky shores that once teemed with a carpet of sea urchins are now distinctly threadbare. The price has rocketed to around £280 per kilogram and the world is being scoured to satisfy this oriental obsession.

As with many aphrodisiacs, the amber roe that is the edible part of the sea urchin turns out to be its sex organs. The five tongues of flesh lining the shell produce the millions of eggs and sperm required for successful aquatic reproduction. Each spawning season, like marine tumbleweed blowing across the sea floor, the sea urchins gather. Releasing a potent sex pheromone, the colony is attracted ever closer together. The pheromone intensity increases until finally it is too much to bear, the colony takes a collective breath and then as one explodes in spectacular simultaneous orgasm and ovulation. The sea becomes a sexual soup of sea urchin effluent. This prodigious fertility is reason enough to finger the sea urchin as an agent provocateur. Combine this saltiness with unusually impressive nutritional statistics and you have a bona fide aphrodisiac all-star.

Sea urchin contains the usual shellfish smorgasbord of libido-enhancing nutrients. Zinc, phosphorus, iodine and potassium are all present and correct in impressive abundance.

In addition to these sex-hormone-supporting minerals, sea urchin contains a rare cannabinoid neurotransmitter called anandamide. As the name suggests, it acts on the brain like cannabis, bringing on intense feelings of pleasure. The scientists who discovered anandamide, quite possibly a little high, named it after the Sanskrit word for bliss, *ananda*. In addition to simply making you feel what a Jamaican might call *irie*, anandamide is released in women at ovulation. This release corresponds to peaks in libido-driving oestrogen and testosterone levels. It is evolution's way of ensuring eggs get fertilised. There is every reason to conclude that for women at least, anandamide is a very direct aphrodisiac. Sea urchin is the only identified food source of anandamide, so for females fulminating with friskiness, simply season with sea hedgehog – truly a woman's best friend. The results from one of my more pleasurable sessions of scientific self-experimentation show that sea urchins are also pretty friendly to men.

In Japan, to best harness its aphrodisiac effect, sea urchin is eaten raw as sashimi or sushi, seasoned with the standard wasabi and soy sauce. Italy is another centre of urchin fancying. In Sardinia, where the rocky coast and crystal waters pulse with spiny life, sea urchin is the principal ingredient in the classic pasta dish *linguine ai ricci di mare*. Raw sea urchin is tossed through linguine flavoured with lemon, chilli, garlic, parsley and olive oil. If this seems like too much trouble, simply spread on toast the way they do in the Shetland Islands of Scotland. If you wish to go gourmand, whisk some raw sea urchin into a hollandaise to set off a superlative seafood brunch of poached eggs and samphire.

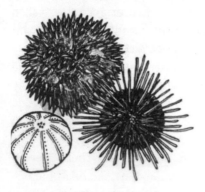

Linguine ai Ricci di Mare

Sea urchins : 10

Dry linguine : 300 g

Extra virgin olive oil (mildly flavoured) : 2 tbsp

Garlic : 1 clove

Red chilli : ½ mild chilli

Lemon : ½

Parsley (finely chopped) : 1 tbsp

Salt and pepper : to taste

Sea urchin, like all seafood, is at its best when at its most fresh. Nothing beats diving for sea urchins and eating them on the rocks then and there. When buying sea urchins, look out for firm spines and a tightly clenched mouth. Avoid any that smell fishy.

Wearing a thick rubber glove, grasp the sea urchin and cut a circle around the mouth orifice. As this comes away it will bring the digestive tract with it – discard both. Scrape out the orange meat with a small teaspoon and strain the liquid from each sea urchin into a bowl.

Cook the linguine as per instructions.

In a pan heat the olive oil, add the garlic crushed into a paste and the finely chopped chilli. Cook for a minute, then add the juice of half a lemon, and the sea urchin meat and juice. Beat together and warm through.

Add the sauce to the pasta and toss with the chopped parsley. Season with sea salt and black pepper.

Eggs Oursinade

Sea urchins : 10
Sun-dried tomato : 4
Freshly squeezed lemon juice : 1 tsp
White vermouth : 1 tsp
Tabasco : a few drops
Hollandaise : 100ml
Eggs (very fresh) : 4
Samphire : 1 large handful
Butter : 1 tbsp
English muffins : 2
Salt and pepper : to taste

Prepare the sea urchins. Add half to a bowl with finely chopped sun-dried tomato, lemon juice, vermouth and Tabasco. Leave to marinate.

Prepare the hollandaise (see artichokes, p84–5 for recipe). Once complete, beat in the remaining sea urchin meat and keep warm.

Poach the very fresh eggs in trembling water (see asparagus, p88–9 for recipe).

Blanch the samphire for 60 seconds in boiling water.

Beat the butter into the marinated sea urchin mix to form a smooth paste.

Toast the muffins, cut them in half and spread with the sea urchin paste.

Place the poached eggs on the muffin halves, spoon over the urchin hollandaise and scatter the plate with the samphire.

Season with salt and freshly ground pepper.

Herbs

BASIL

The risqué Victorian adventurer Sir Richard Burton observed that basil 'unless it is warmed by the fingers, emits no perfume'; the old rogue goes on to add, 'much like a woman'. And it seems that since antiquity women and basil have been the best of friends. A Roman woman would dust her bosom with dried basil to ensure her lover's lasting affection; the scent was well known to drive men wild. A theory also subscribed to by Italian prostitutes who centuries later would smear themselves with basil oil to attract punters; it remains unclear whether this was indeed to drive men wild or perhaps to mask less savoury odours.

By way of contrast, in India, holy basil or *tulsi* is the preserve of the devout, who regard it as the manifestation of the goddess Tulasi. Hindu legend tells of Lord Vishnu tricking Tulasi into some extramarital rumpy pumpy by masquerading as her husband. Legend is delicately unspecific regarding the exact moment Vishnu's ruse was uncovered, but uncovered it was. Mortified by her infidelity, Tulasi promptly threw herself on to a bonfire and was burnt to a cinder. From the smoking ashes of her burnt body sprung up a profusion of basil bushes and Vishnu, unrepentant but impressed by this woman's fidelity, declared that Tulasi should be worshipped for her faithfulness and that the herb *tulsi* should represent her. Thus holy basil became a symbol of love and fidelity for millions of Hindus.

It is unlikely that you would ever eat enough basil for it to have a significant aphrodisiac effect from its nutritional composition. Any bedroom impulses must therefore stem from basil's fragrance and flavour, which come from its peculiarly high concentration of essential oils. In modern aromatherapy basil is used as a mental and emotional pick-me-up. It dispels melancholy, sharpens the senses and induces a euphoric, giddy feeling; from this description it sounds all too likely that basil does indeed put one in the mood for a little rough and tumble. A more scientific study offers additional support, showing that basil, sweet basil and holy basil all contain the compound eugenol. Without getting too technical, eugenol dilates one's blood vessels. This increases blood flow to one's extremities, turning the diminutive wee man into an incredible hulk. What better way to enliven these unmentionable extremities than a 'relaxing' cup of herbal basil tea before bedtime?

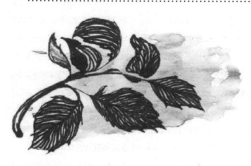

Tulsi Tea
Holy basil is a wild variant of common basil; it is available from pretty much all oriental stores and is great substituted for common basil in all cooked dishes. To make Tulsi tea take

a good sprig of fresh holy basil, the zest of half an orange, a few cardamom pods and a spoonful of honey. Place all the ingredients except the honey in a pot and fill with boiling water. Leave to infuse for 5 minutes and add the honey to taste. Sweet dreams.

MINT

There are over twenty-five varieties of mint. Although they all smell and taste similarly fresh and fragrant their aphrodisiac effects can be polar opposites. History has been correspondingly confused over mint's aphrodisiac credentials.

In the fourth century BC medical maestro Hippocrates gave mint the most dismal diagnosis, declaring that it diluted sperm, weakened erections and tired the body. Aristotle's opinion was the exact opposite. He thought mint such an aphrodisiac that he formally advised Alexander the Great to forbid his troops from drinking mint tea on campaign lest their minds wandered to less warlike activities. As long as Hippocrates was railing against spearmint and Aristotle championing peppermint, they could both have been right.

Modern medical research has revealed spearmint to be quite the party pooper when it comes to adult activities. Spearmint tea is effective as a treatment for hirsutism in women. Although bearded ladies are not my particular cup of tea, neither is the chemical action that banishes the bristles. Spearmint has anti-androgenic properties and reduces the level of free testosterone in the body. Bio-available testosterone sounds the charge for carnal conquest so this state of affairs is far from ideal. Bearded bon viveurs hell bent on bed bouncing should give it a wide berth.

Peppermint smells much like spearmint but has very different chemical components. Its essential oil is up to 70 per cent menthol, compared with the paltry ½ per cent in spearmint oil. This difference makes all the difference. Menthol behaves like capsaicin in chilli, triggering the body's heat sensors. Whereas chilli fools the body into thinking it is hot, peppermint produces a cooling sensation. The body responds to this temperature threat by dilating blood vessels and raising the heart rate. This elevated state of metabolism mirrors that of arousal, allowing seamless transition from numbing minty chill to hot tingling passion.

It is a crying shame that the mint most commonly used in cooking is spearmint. The sprig with your new potatoes, scenting peas and slathering roast lamb may be delicious but is decidedly unhelpful in propagating romance. Say a sad sayonara to Mojitos and mint juleps and a questionable hello to crème de menthe. Peppermint is most widely used in confectionary and ice cream. The gastronome can at least give a small cheer for after-dinner mint fondants and mint choc chip.

Peppermint Fondants

Egg : 1
Icing sugar : 400 g + extra for dusting
Lemon juice : a squeeze
Peppermint extract : 1 tsp
Bitter dark chocolate
(70% cocoa solids) : 200 g

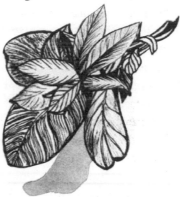

*Separate the egg white from
the yolk and whisk it in a clean
bowl until it forms soft peaks.*

*Gradually whisk sifted icing
sugar into the egg white and
finally whisk in the lemon juice
and peppermint extract. The mix
should be a thick paste. Taste the fondant mix and if you want a
stronger mint kick add a little more peppermint.*

*Dust a board with icing sugar and roll out the fondant mix to
a thickness of under ½ cm. Place the rolled fondant on a sheet of
non-stick parchment paper and allow to air dry for a few hours.*

*Once firm, use a sharp knife to cut out neat 4 cm squares.
Put the fondants in the freezer for 20 minutes to firm them up
completely, ready to be dipped in chocolate.*

*Break the chocolate into pieces and melt in a pan set
over simmering water. Once melted, one by one immerse the
fondants in the chocolate. Delicately fish them out with two forks
and place on non-stick parchment paper to set.*

ROCKET

For those fond of certainties rocket is a little confusing. It hovers mysteriously between herb and salad, and I am never quite sure whether it prefers the names arugula or roquette to rocket. If what's-its-name is a salad it is an unusual one. According to legend, lettuce stifles the libido whereas rocket does the exact opposite.

In classical antiquity, rocket was sacred to the god Priapus. The son of beautiful Aphrodite and dissolute Dionysus, Priapus has the most erotic pedigree and is best known for his large, ever-ready erection. Rocket was planted at the rural shrines dedicated to Priapus. It was widely believed that a quick graze on its peppery leaves would have male members standing at full attention, swollen with devout desire. In Dioscorides's authoritative *Pharmacopeia* of herbal remedies, raw rocket and its seeds are formally fingered as powerful aphrodisiacs. Rocket's reputation survived the sack of Rome, thriving in subsequent Spanish Visigoth culture. The Archbishop of Seville, St Isidore, is often referred to as the last scholar of the ancient world. His saintly seventh-century mind was not above observing the rocket effect. In his *Etymologiae* (the first Christian encyclopaedia) Isidore writes that 'rocket is, so to speak, inflammatory, since it has burning properties and, if consumed frequently in the diet arouses the sexual appetite'.

A few hundred years later, the Church took a much dimmer view of such properties. They banned rocket from monastic diets and their general disapproval led to rocket largely disappearing from the cuisines of Europe. Italy was the notable exception. The recent popularity of rustic Italian food has seen rocket restored to global gastronomic favour.

Rocket's hot, peppery taste is the fuel for its aphrodisiac reputation. Just as chilli, pepper, mustard, horseradish and peppermint trip our heat-sensitive defence system, so does rocket. The distinctive pungent taste of raw rocket sensitises the mouth, raises the metabolism and dilates blood vessels. This spirited state of affairs puts one in a decidedly frisky mood; a sniff of stimulation and you will be rampant as a randy rabbit. The glucosinolates responsible for rocket's fiery frisson are defused by cooking. Restrict culinary adventure to the raw experience. Tossed with olive oil and sprinkled with shavings of Parmesan, it makes a salad sophisticated enough for any occasion. Rocket's punchy flavour stands up well to the boldness of beef, its heat a delightful and necessary counterpoint to the raw reality of beef carpaccio. The same idea works to more dramatic effect with beef tataki rolls filled with rocket and curls of buttery avocado – if you are feeling flash you can substitute the avocado with curls of chilled foie gras to excellent effect and no doubt ecstatic approval all round.

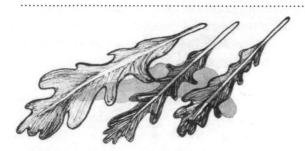

Rocket, Avocado and Beef Tataki Rolls

Beef fillet (tail piece) : 250 g
Vegetable oil : 1 tbsp
Sesame oil : 1 tsp
Balsamic vinegar : 1 tbsp
Honey : 1 tsp
Tabasco : a few drops
Rocket : 50 g
Avocado : 1
Chives : 4
Toasted sesame seeds : 1 tbsp

Brush the beef with the vegetable oil. Heat a heavy-based non-stick frying pan and when it is very hot, sear the meat on all sides. Wrap the seared meat in cling film and refrigerate for a few hours.

Mix the sesame oil with the balsamic vinegar, honey and Tabasco to create a glaze. Cut the chives into 8 cm lengths.

Slice the beef very thinly and brush one side of each slice with the sesame balsamic glaze. Place a few leaves of rocket, a curl of

avocado and two pieces of chive down the centre of each slice
and wrap up to form a loose roll.

Place each roll on a large rocket leaf and sprinkle each one
with a few toasted sesame seeds.

....

ROSE

A bon viveur embraces all things floral. Unimaginative yet
effective, the well-chosen posy delights all but the most
disagreeable. When it comes to charming the ladies, roses are
the most attentive, witty and debonair of suitors. Men are
equally at sea; the scent of rose bewitches and bamboozles. It
is the essence of unbridled femininity, mysterious and utterly
compelling. The perfume wafts into the kitchen. Rose is used to
scent and flavour food, adding a seductive edge of languorous
sensuality.

The rose has been a symbol of love since antiquity. In ancient
Egypt it was sacred to Isis, the goddess of motherhood, magic
and fertility. Greek legend attributes the rose's romantic origins
to a veritable dream team of divinity. Chloris, the goddess of
flowers, found a favourite nymph dead in a woodland clear-
ing. Grieving, she decided to turn her into the most beautiful
flower the world had ever seen. She enlisted Aphrodite to give
the rose beauty; Dionysus added nectar and beguiling scent and
the three Graces gave charm, brightness and joy. Zephyr, the
gentle west wind, chased away the clouds and Apollo, the sun
god, shone and made the rose bloom. Bees attracted to the rose's
heady perfume proceeded to sting a passing Eros. The dashing

deity of desire, somewhat miffed, drew his bow and let fly with a hail of arrows. He missed his target and the arrows struck the rose bush, leaving sharp thorns along its stem.

The ancients took the erotic origins to heart. In Egypt, ever eager for aphrodisiac advantage, Cleopatra carpeted her pleasure palace with rose petals. When she seduced Mark Antony it is said they lay an inch thick over the floor of her bedchamber. The Emperor Nero, *dissolutus maximus* of ancient Rome, took rose fancying to extreme levels. At home to decadence and debauchery, he lounged on pillows filled with rose petals, drank rose-flavoured wine, ate rose pudding for afters and cavorted naked in rose-perfumed pools. The Arab world was equally impressed. Clay tablets from the ancient temple of Ur, in modern-day Iraq, document Baghdad's infatuation with roses. The sultan's clearly extensive harem got through a mighty 30,000 jars of rose water a year. In 1718, Lady Mary Wortley Montagu, wife to the British ambassador in Istanbul, wrote of the secret rose language of the harem. Lovers were not allowed to express their love openly in the harems of the Ottoman Empire. Instead they exchanged roses. A furled red rose signalled budding desire, an open red rose was more forward, stating that one was full of love and lust. An open white rose asked, 'Will you love me?' whilst an open yellow rose pleaded, 'Do you still love me?'

It was in Ottoman Istanbul that the rose found its most celebrated culinary use. The sultan Abdul Hamid I commissioned his master sweet-maker to devise a confection to wow the jaded palates of his wives and mistresses. In 1776 Hadji Bekir created *rahat lokum*, a candy of set rose syrup dusted in sugar.

The harem was agog. In the eighteenth century it was exported to England, renamed with all the exoticism of the East as Turkish delight.

The tradition, scent and physical beauty of the rose are all achingly romantic. The psychological associations and heady sensual aroma are more than enough to suffuse a dish with aphrodisiac appeal. It is pleasing, however, to find scientific support. Studies at the Smell and Taste Treatment and Research Foundation in Chicago have recently found that the scent of roses increases olfactory-evoked nostalgia. Happy memories and loving occasions spring back to life – the warm fuzzy glow to start an amorous fire.

Rose is a sweet, heady fragrance. In gastronomy it only really works in desserts and sweetened drinks. A sticky sponge pudding scented with rose syrup and drenched in vanilla custard would surely invoke the spirit of Nero's decadent feasts. The sweet-toothed Iranians are passionate about rose-water ice cream. This combination works particularly well. The coolness counteracts and sharpens the potentially cloying sweetness of the rose. In North Africa, rose is often used in the savoury spice mix *ras el hanout*. Here the sweetness of rose is balanced by the kick of chilli and pepper. In Turkish delight the addition of lemon juice does the same job, tempering the rose with sharp acidity. A delicately set cube of Turkish delight melts on the tongue with intoxicating effect. Eyes glaze and mouths slip open. Unleash said effect with this surprisingly simple recipe.

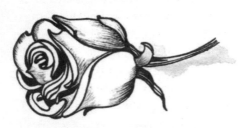

Rose and Pomegranate Turkish Delight

Water : 250 ml
Cornflour : 35 g + 1 tsp
Cream of tartar : ½ tsp
Caster sugar : 200 g
Freshly squeezed lemon juice : 1 tbsp
Freshly squeezed pomegranate juice : 1 tbsp
Rose water : 2 tbsp
Icing sugar : 3 tbsp

In a small pan mix 150 ml of water with the cornflour and cream of tartar. Whisk together, then heat until the mixture has thickened.

In another pan heat the caster sugar with remaining 100 ml of water, the lemon juice and pomegranate juice. You need pure pomegranate juice for this recipe, so it is best to squeeze a fresh fruit. Heat to 115°C (soft ball stage on a sugar thermometer).

Remove from the heat and steadily add the cornflour mixture to the sugar syrup, whisking furiously to combine. Return to the heat and continue to cook until the mix reaches 120°C.

Remove from the heat and allow to cool slightly. Add the

rose water and stir to combine – as all rose water has different strengths it is best to do this a teaspoon at a time, tasting as you go.

Pour the mixture into a silicone ice-cube tray (or a deep baking tray lined with parchment paper). Allow to cool, then chill for 2 hours to complete the setting process. Turn the pieces out of the ice-cube tray, or if set in a baking tray, use a sharp knife to cut the Turkish Delight into chunky cubes.

Finally toss in a bowl containing the icing sugar mixed with a teaspoon of cornflour. If the idea of a contrasting crispy coating floats your boat, toss in crushed toasted almond flakes or pulverised pistachio nuts.

Spices

CHILLI

Pleasure and pain are at the heart of chilli's aphrodisiac reputation. Like the stinging crack of a dominatrix's crop, the hit of too much chilli is without question a painful experience. Tender derrières and sensitive tongues will be equally on fire. I have often wondered why it is that the body rewards such masochism with the warm embrace of confused arousal.

Psychologist Paul Rozin puts forward the theory of 'con strained risk'. The exhilaration you feel riding a roller coaster is enjoyable only because your fear is unfounded. Your body believes it is in an extreme situation but you know you are perfectly safe. You can enjoy the rush of adrenaline recognising that you aren't going to have to either fight or flee. The same principle applies to pain. The sensation of pain is the body defending itself from harmful threats. The pain from a hot curry, or a playful spanking, triggers a slightly different defence mechanism but again there is no real threat to bodily well-being. The sudden rush of pleasure-giving endorphins is designed to anaesthetise pain, allowing an injured animal to make good its escape to safety. As there is no real danger to evade, you can focus on pleasure instead. The feel-good raised pulse, dilated blood vessels and sweating of the chilli buzz are sensations shared with the physiology of sexual desire. When there is no escaping to be done, the confused mind defaults to the sexual response, kindling a libidinous inferno.

Those with steam coming out of their ears will argue that the pain they feel is very real indeed. The solutions are simple: milk or moderation. Cold milk is the most effective way to extinguish a chilli fire. Milk's casein proteins have a detergent effect on the capsaicin in chilli, washing away unwanted heat but leaving that sensitive glow. Moderation is less likely to set fire to your libido but then again it is also less likely to douse your shirt in perspiration and turn you into a sweaty mess. A little sweat is quite enough to send forth your come-hither perfume of sexual pheromones. The effect is likely to be undermined if you need to towel yourself down. Similarly, dilated pupils, a slight flush and a pouty plumping of the lips signals sexual interest far more effectively than scarlet-chested, wide-eyed staring.

Chilli evolved its unique heat as a biological defence mechanism. Deciding that birds were the best way of scattering their seed, chillis devised the burning compound capsaicin as a way of deterring seed-crushing mammals from eating their fruit. Unlike mammals, birds are immune to capsaicin – a characteristic exploited today in the chilli-treated seed that birdies use to confound feeder-thieving Squirrel Nutkins. Unlike us, squirrels don't know that pain is in the mind and they leave well alone.

The use of chilli as an aphrodisiac is long-standing. In its native Central America, the fortifying hot chocolate widely drunk as an aphrodisiac was seasoned with the sharp smack to the system of fresh chilli. Montezuma, the conquistadored Aztec king, was a chilli-chocoholic. Whether his daily tangle with his team of concubines was cause or effect is unknown – either way he is said to have drunk fifty glasses a day. Migrating to Europe with returning explorers, chilli soon spread across the warmer parts of the world. In Indian and Chinese traditional medicine, chilli is used to heat up a frigid metabolism. It is employed to boost the similar concepts of vatta and yang, which are gauges of libido.

If you also want to re-calibrate libidos upwards, chilli can be just the ticket. As discussed already, its aphrodisiac appeal lies in applying the correct dose. For maximum gratification you want heat levels to hover just under bearable. To ensure there are no unscheduled explosions, the prudent bon viveur adds his chilli at the end of cooking as if seasoning with salt. Removing the seeds and scraping away the fiery inner membrane and pith also allows for a larger margin of error. Sugar syrup comes a close second to milk as a calming balm for a burning mouth. Thai sweet chilli dipping sauce uses this to great effect allowing the enjoyment of more heat with less burn. Incredibly versatile, it makes a fantastic dressing for the fusion dish of squid ink spaghetti with tiger prawns, bok choi and Szechuan pepper. Less glamorous but equally fusion is the midnight snack of toast, cream cheese, sweet chilli sauce and grated mature cheddar. Similarly simple is another oriental favourite: Vietnamese green mango and crab summer rolls come with a sidekick of liquid fire in their classic chilli and vinegar accompaniment – almost hallucinatory, strangely addictive but undoubtedly arousing.

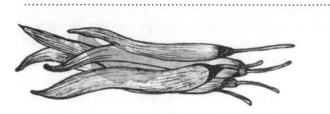

Green Mango and Crab Summer Rolls with Chilli Dipping Sauce

SUMMER ROLLS

Green mango : 1 small mango
Spring onion : 3
Mint : ½ tbsp
Coriander : a small handful
Thai basil : a small handful
Rice vermicelli : 80 g
White crabmeat : 100 g
Bean sprouts : a handful
Black sesame seeds : 1 tsp
Toasted white sesame seeds : 1 tsp
Toasted sesame oil : 1 tsp
Ricepaper pancakes : 6

Grate the mango and finely slice the spring onion, mint, basil and coriander.

Cook the rice vermicelli as per instructions, then refresh under cold water.

Mix the vermicelli, herbs, mango and onion with the crabmeat, bean sprouts, sesame seeds and sesame oil.

One by one, dip the ricepaper pancakes for 5 seconds in tepid water then place a line of filling along the middle of the pancake. Fold each end in and roll tightly into 4 cm cylinders.

Serve cut in half on the diagonal.

CHILLI DIPPING SAUCE
Bird's eye chilli : 2
Lime : 1
Fish sauce : 2 tbsp
Rice vinegar : 2 tbsp
Rice wine : 2 tbsp
Palm sugar : 1 tbsp

Finely chop the chilli and zest the lime.

Place all the ingredients in a small pan and over a gentle heat stir until the sugar dissolves.

Taste and add additional salt, sweetness or sharpness as required. The flavour should be a balance between the saltiness of the fish sauce, the heat of the chilli, the sweetness of the sugar and sharpness of the vinegar.

Serve in a shallow dipping bowl.

GARLIC

Garlic is the ringleader of a pretty pungent aphrodisiac gang. This foul-mouthed crew includes onions, shallots, leeks and chives. Accused of inciting desire, these outlaws are unwelcome at Buddhist monasteries and among Hindu Brahmins.

Asceticism is anathema to the bon viveur. Clasp these renegades to your bosom and let romance blossom under the stinking rose's sensory benediction.

I like to think the stinking rose refers to garlic's base aphrodisiac appeal. Certainly the ancient Greeks, who first coined the phrase, were firm believers. It was part of the daily diet: athletes gobbled it before Olympic competition, soldiers likewise before martial feats. The maverick medicos Hippocrates and Galen both agreed that garlic gave potency a good poking. The tradition survives to the present day. Garlic is Greece's most popular aphrodisiac, popping up everywhere from the creamy tang of tzatziki to the garlicky potato paste of skordalia, and pretty much everywhere in between. On the Ionian Islands, widowers who remarry are fortified for marital manliness with a pre-wedding feast of garlic-based dishes.

India's Ayurvedic traditions are in absolute agreement. More mature men whose sexual moon may be waning are directed to garlic's get-up-and-go. More generally, it is recommended wholesale as a sexual tonic for almost any sexual misfortune: impotency from overindulgence to nervous exhaustion from dissipating habits. Garlic is classed as both *rajasic* and *tamasic*, fuelling passion and ignorance. It rouses the body and suppresses the mind. Understandably, yogis who have taken a vow of celibacy rarely test their resolve with a nice aioli. Those of us who are vow-free are advised to forget themselves, enjoy that aioli and revel in the rousing.

This is no mystic mumbo-jumbo. Garlic is scientifically proven to bring on the lover man. It not only boosts circulation but more importantly stimulates the release of nitric oxide.

Nitric oxide is the messenger boy of arousal, the signal for downstairs to unleash a man's Moby Dick. The willingness to wield one's hormonal harpoon is also boosted. Experiments on rats show that garlic and a high-protein diet significantly increase testosterone levels. If ever an excuse was needed for a steak slathered in garlic butter, now you have it.

The only cloud on garlic's aphrodisiac horizon is the spectre of halitosis. More than any other failing, I find it hard to overlook bad breath. Holding your nose is no way to make love. The smell of raw garlic on the breath is strong but not unpleasant. The true garlic breath needs time to mature. As garlic is digested it produces allyl methyl sulphide, a noxious-smelling sulphurous compound that cannot be digested. Instead it is absorbed into the blood from where it is finally excreted from the lungs and skin, causing the telltale fetid breath and rank sweat of yesterday's garlic binge. Some claim parsley is an effective remedy. Although it hides the initial blast of raw garlic, parsley does little for the subsequent miasma. Milk, however, goes some way to stopping the rot. Milk proteins absorb this sulphurous compound quite effectively, allowing you to quietly kick garlic out the back door having had your fun.

Garlic is extremely versatile in the kitchen. Crushed raw garlic presents a ferociously feisty proposition. The crushing process activates garlic's allicin, which is primarily responsible for its strong flavour. Salt, parsley and lemon attenuate its strength but a little still goes a long way. Briefly cooking garlic mellows it greatly. Roasting whole bulbs produces an almost entirely different flavour, rich and sweet with scarcely a trace of its raw fieriness. Although cooking may reduce garlic's aphrodisiac efficiency, in this instance the gourmet is going to have the final say. A roast garlic and butter bean soup flavoured with Parmesan is a silky, sensual delight. Drizzle some melted garlic butter over the top to provide contrast to its civilised restraint. If it is groin you are principally after, unleash some machismo on a juicy steak with a feisty garlic, fresh herb and anchovy *beurre maison*. Head off halitosis by washing it down with a glass of milk.

Garlic *Beurre Maison*

Garlic : 3 fat cloves
Sea salt : ½ tsp
Salted anchovy : 2 fillets
Butter : 75 g
Parsley : 1 tbsp
Rosemary : 1 tsp
Black pepper : ½ tsp

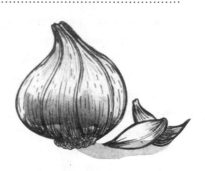

Remove the skin from your garlic cloves. Using a serrated dining knife scrape away at each clove until it is a mush. Using the salt as an abrasive, scrape the knife repeatedly over the mush until the garlic becomes a very smooth viscous paste.

Finely chop the anchovy fillets, then work them into the garlic paste in the same way as before. They should be as thoroughly combined as is possible. You could use anchovy paste or Gentleman's Relish if you have these to hand.

Warm the butter slightly, then work it into the garlic paste.

Finely chop the herbs and grind the pepper, then mix into the butter.

Transfer the butter to a piece of cling film and roll into a sausage about 2.5 cm in diameter. Place the butter in the fridge to chill thoroughly.

The butter is now ready for your steak. Cut a 1 cm round from your butter log. Pop it on the steak immediately prior to serving, so it melts at the table. The butter can also be used to make garlic bread and is fantastic worked into a chicken before roasting. Asparagus loves it, as do roast scallops and snails.

Roast Garlic and Butter Bean Soup

Garlic : 2 large heads
Salt : to taste
Olive oil : 2 tsp
Butter beans : 400 g (1 can)
Chicken stock : 500 ml
Bay leaf : 2
Thyme : 1 small sprig
Clove : 2
Peppercorn : 2
Butter : 50 g
Parmesan : 2 tbsp grated
Double cream : 100 ml
Parsley : 1 tsp

Preheat the oven to 180°C.

With a sharp knife cut across the top of both heads of garlic – about one third down from the pointed end. Discard the top third and season the bottom part of each bulb with a pinch of sea salt and a teaspoon of olive oil. Loosely wrap each head in foil and place in the preheated oven to cook for one hour. Once cooked the garlic should be very soft, sweet and oozing with mellow flavour.

Remove the butter beans from the can and rinse under cold running water. If you want the smoothest, silkiest texture to the soup remove the skin from the butter beans too.

Place the rinsed, skinned beans in a large pan with the chicken stock and all of the herbs and spices except the parsley. Bring to the boil then turn the heat down, cover with a lid and simmer gently for 20 minutes.

Strain the beans, taking care to reserve the infused chicken stock. Remove the herbs and spices from the beans and discard. Place the beans in a blender with the butter and squeeze in the flesh from the roast garlic heads. Add two thirds of the chicken stock and blend until very smooth.

The blended soup should have the consistency of double cream – add the remaining stock gradually until you have the desired thickness.

Pass the soup through a fine sieve back into the pan. Stir in the Parmesan and the double cream. Taste and season if required with salt. The soup will benefit from being left overnight for the flavours to mature but this is by no means essential.

Finely chop the parsley so it is almost like dust.

Pour the soup into bowls. Put the parsley in a sieve and shake over the soup to give it an even green dusting. Serve with crusty bread and a rich white Burgundy.

GINGER

Ginger is the panacea of the spice world. Chinese and Ayurvedic medicine regard this fiery root as a healing gift from the gods. It can clear a cold, soothe an upset stomach, still nausea and dry diarrhoea. The list goes on. Cancer, arthritis, circulation – there is almost nothing that cannot be cured with ginger's healing heat. It goes almost without saying that ginger is also an aphrodisiac.

Ginger's groin-warming goodness was first documented in the first century AD. Graeco-Roman physician Dioscorides recommends it as stimulating to the male organ. In the tenth century the illustrious Arab doctor Avicenna credits it with 'increasing lustful yearnings'. Five hundred years later, the famed mediaeval medical school in Salerno was advising ageing romantics to 'eat ginger, and you will love and be loved as in your youth'. If feeling extreme, our autumnal lovers could take things several steps further. Figging is the distinctly fringe practice of gingering a basement orifice. It was originally devised to keep horses' tails high on parade; enquiring Victorian minds decided to try it for themselves and found it was surprisingly good, though probably not morally so. The initial burn apparently gives way to unbridled desire.

Modern medicine is generally impressed by ginger's curative claims. Its aphrodisiac reputation is equally well founded. Ginger's zingy flavour and sharp heat come from three volatile oils: gingerol, zingerone and shogaol. Subtler cousins of the chilli kick, ginger's active ingredients stimulate the body in much the same way. They trigger sensory receptors designed to detect heat and physical abrasion. The body experiences a burning sensation and yelps. Biological defence mechanisms quickly kick in to put out the problem. Pulse rates race and blood vessels dilate in a coordinated effort to protect the damaged tissue. Anticipating ongoing anguish, the body also issues a stream of soothing endorphins, papering over the pain with pleasure. This combination is a ringer for arousal. As ginger's burn subsides quickly, these warming effects can turn suddenly to wide-eyed arousal.

Ginger's aromatic and earthy, citrus heat tickles taste buds as well as biological defence mechanisms. The intense oriental flavours of ginger, chilli and garlic are the cornerstone of Indian and Chinese cooking. The base for almost every Indian curry, they are equally ubiquitous in the broths and stir-fries of China. The Japanese eat ginger pickled, in between bites of sushi. In Europe and America, ginger is all about baking. As fresh ginger would rot before reaching Europe, it was always imported in its dried and ground form. Ground ginger was used to spice biscuits, bread, cookies, cakes and drinks. The first gingerbread men were English, appearing spontaneously in Elizabeth I's court. Ginger beer popped up in the seventeenth century. English taverns put out pots of ground ginger as a condiment. Some experimental punter put a pinch in his pint and the rest is history.

As with most ingredients, ginger is best fresh. Although ground ginger is twice as hot as fresh ginger, the fresh variety provides a far more exhilarating blast of upfront flavour. The kick is pretty keen in a warming glass of ginger tea – black tea spiced with a couple of slices of fresh ginger and sweetened with honey. When it comes to dining I rarely get past the classic Chinese combination of beef and ginger. Their strong warming flavours are a match made in heaven. Rouse passions and save money with a crispy beef and ginger stir-fry that craftily stretches one steak across two mouths.

....

Crispy Beef with Ginger Fries

Rump steak : 250 g
Garlic : 2 cloves
Red chilli : 1
Rice wine : 2 tbsp
Dark soy sauce : 2 tbsp
Toasted sesame oil : 2 tbsp
Honey : 2 tbsp
Ginger root : 100 g
Fine green beans : 100 g
Spring onion : 100 g
Cornflour : 100 g
Salt : a large pinch
Chinese five-spice : 1 tbsp
Egg : 1
Vegetable oil : 100 ml

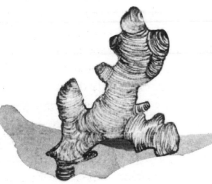

Cut the steak into thin strips. Work across the grain of the meat, ideally producing strips that are 5 cm long by about 1 cm wide and ½ cm thick.

Crush the garlic with the back of a knife and a little table salt. Mix this paste with finely chopped chilli, rice wine, soy sauce, toasted sesame oil and honey. Pour this marinade over the beef strips, cover and leave to marinate for at least 2 hours.

Meanwhile peel the ginger and cut into matchsticks. Top and tail the fine beans (alternatively you could use thin asparagus or purple sprouting broccoli sliced in half lengthways). Finely slice the spring onion on the diagonal.

Remove the beef from the marinade, and allow to air dry. Reserve the marinade.

Mix the cornflour with salt and five-spice. Beat the egg. Coat the beef strips in beaten egg, then toss in the cornflour mix until well coated.

Heat the vegetable oil in a wok or large heavy saucepan. When it is very hot, add half the beef and fry for about 2 minutes until golden brown. Remove and keep warm whilst frying the remaining beef.

After frying the beef allow the oil to become very hot again. Toss the ginger matchsticks in the spiced cornflour, shake off any excess flour and then deep-fry for about 30 seconds until golden brown. Remove and keep warm.

Reduce the amount of oil in the pan to just 1 tablespoon.

Stir-fry the green beans for 30 seconds, then add the sliced spring onion and stir-fry for 10 seconds longer. Finally add the marinade.

Return the crispy beef and ginger fries to the wok. Toss to combine and serve immediately with steamed rice, and bok choi dressed with oyster sauce.

MUSTARD

Although mustard seeds have been used as a spice since time immemorial, it was the road-building Romans who invented modern mustard. They pounded mustard seeds with unfermented grape juice or must. The resulting paste was so fiery that it became known as burning must, *mustum ardens*, and so via Chinese whispers to mustard. It was massively popular in Roman times, an essential condiment for meat and fish that sat on almost every dining table. One of the reasons it was so popular was a deep-seated belief that mustard inflamed the senses. Pliny the Elder wrote that 'with a few spoonfuls of mustard, a cold and lazy woman can become an ideal wife'. Somehow I don't think Pliny is referring to housework.

By the Middle Ages, mustard's aphrodisiac reputation was sufficiently entrenched for the Church to banish it from monkish tables, fearing sexual mayhem in the monastery. Attempting just such a scenario, frigid Danish dames thawed their dainties with a potion of mustard, mint and ginger. I assume only the extremely keen applied this externally. The Chinese had of course known all this for millennia. Due to mustard's warming properties, Chinese medicine had long regarded its seeds as a powerful aphrodisiac yang tonic.

When it comes to divining its aphrodisiac effect the Chinese were almost certainly on the right track. To say mustard is warming can be something of an understatement. A strong English variety thrashes the tongue, sears the nose and sets eyes watering. Then as suddenly as it arrived the sensory crisis is over, leaving an invigorated diner with tingling senses.

Biologically, mustard's molten assault triggers the release of soothing, euphoric endorphins. It also quickens the pulse, dilates the blood vessels and generally raises one's metabolism. Research from Oxford has shown mustard to boost metabolism as effectively as ephedrine, speeding it by as much as 25 per cent for several hours. The symptoms are a simulacrum for sexual arousal. Mustard simply bamboozles the body into desire. The active ingredient, allyl isothiocyanate, is also responsible for the kick in horseradish, wasabi and rocket.

The heat in mustard depends greatly on how it is made. Bizarrely, the most important factor is the temperature of the liquid mixed with the ground mustard seed. Cold water produces the fieriest paste whilst the warm dilutions of Dijon produce a milder, more refined mustard. Cooked out in a sauce, the fire is all but extinguished. The varieties of seed also play a part. White mustard seed is responsible for the tongue lashing. Black mustard (actually juncea) rises up the nose.

The bon viveur should approach mustard with a little caution. Although the aphrodisiac effect is keenest with crying-strength mustard, too much is certain to swamp the finer points of a delicate dish. At strength, it sings most sweetly with simple dishes of seasoned pork. A strong smoked ham basks in the heat of a good mustard, whilst a hot dog sits up and begs for the stuff. The gutsy flavours of roast beef and smoked fish similarly stand up and flourish in mustard's potentially overbearing company. Although rarely attempted, making your own mustard is surprisingly simple and can provide new gastronomic heights to this ubiquitous condiment. Set pulses racing with a personally prepared cider and celery mustard. Quite flash, the apple and celery notes complement pork perfectly. It is guaranteed to impress your sausage.

....

Cider and Celery Banger Mustard

Black mustard seeds : 100 g
Yellow mustard seeds : 100 g
Coriander seed : ½ tsp
Turmeric : ½ tsp
Celery seeds : 1 tsp
Dried thyme : 1 tsp
Sharp apple juice : 150 ml
Sweet cider : 150 ml
Mustard powder : 1 tbsp
Cider vinegar : 100 ml
Sea salt

The main advantage in making your own mustard is its freshness. Unlike commercial mustards, no vinegar or salt is required for preservation. It is used solely for flavour and in much reduced quantities.

In a dry pan heat the mustard, coriander, turmeric and celery seeds for a few minutes to activate their flavours.

Pour the seeds into a pestle and mortar and crush until very fine.

Pour the resulting powder into a fine sieve. Shake and stir until all the fine particles pass through the sieve and only the larger pieces of seed husk remain. Place this powder with the dried thyme in a bowl and cover with the apple juice and cider. Let the mustard absorb the moisture overnight.

Add the mustard powder to the mix and half the cider vinegar. Leave to stand for 20 minutes, then transfer to a food processor and blend until the mustard is the desired consistency.

Leave to stand for a further 3 hours, add some more vinegar if it is too thick, then blend again.

Season to taste with the remaining vinegar and salt.

If you want a smoother mustard, pass it through the finest sieve you have to remove any remaining husks.

Store for a week before using. Refrigerated, it will keep for months.

....

NUTMEG

Every banana-skin-toking schoolboy knows that nutmeg has narcotic properties and is mildly hallucinogenic. It can be smoked, snorted or eaten. Getting baked on nutmeg is described as a euphoric state somewhere between waking and dreaming. In the 1940s it inspired saxophonist Charlie Bird Parker's improvised flights of jazz fancy. Malcolm X was another nutmeg narco. Not quite on the level of $E=mc^2$, in Charlestown gaol he devised the stoner's equation 1 x nutmeg = 4 x marijuana reefer. Narcotic effect is no guarantee of aphrodisiac ecstacy but it certainly marks nutmeg out for closer inspection.

Formally known as *myristica fragans*, nutmeg is the seed of a tropical evergreen tree that until the 1800s grew exclusively on the Banda Islands of Indonesia. Around the seed is a lacy red coating. This is mace, nutmeg's milder-tasting cousin. As nutmeg was traded further and further from its remote origins it developed a varied aphrodisiac following. The Unani medical tradition of Arabia and India considers nutmeg a warming tonic for fortifying the male libido. In China and Zanzibar it is women who feel nutmeg's aphrodisiac effect. It is a vital ingredient in a Zanzibar bride's pre-wedding porridge. The brides say that it 'makes them loose' – whether this is literal or metaphorical is unclear. In Europe, nutmeg sparked a not insignificant war between the Portuguese, Dutch and British. All wanted control of this desirable spice and its lucrative trade. Nutmeg's external aphrodisiac effect was noted. In seventeenth-century England, maverick master of physick, William Salmon, recommends nutmeg oil on the nether regions. A quick polish with an oily rag and the sexual engine roars into action.

Inquisitive scientists support nutmeg's aphrodisiac credentials. An experiment in India has proved that male rats dosed with nutmeg extract display an increase in both libido and potency. The active ingredient in nutmeg is the compound myristicin. Comprising about 4 per cent of nutmeg's essential oil, myristicin is a weak monoamine oxidase inhibitor. For the uninitiated, what are known in the trade as MAOIs block the oxidisation of monoamines such as dopamine, serotonin, adrenaline and phenylethylamine. The result is higher levels of these pleasurable libido-enhancing chemicals swilling round the brain, tickling away at the brain's bonk spot. Dr Alan Hirsch in his smell studies found that the aroma of pumpkin pie is one of the sexiest scents for both men and women. Nutmeg is the key spice in this American homey classic, providing yet more evidence that it is not only narcotic but rather erotic.

If you want to fly the nutmeg high you are best off with its essential oil. Dip a cigarette in the oil, light up and wreathe yourself in fragrant smoke. Eating the spice is effective but the bumper dose and slightly queasy, twenty-four-hour trip may not be to everyone's taste. Enjoying nutmeg's aphrodisiac effect is more mainstream. Much less nutmeg is needed – a heavily seasoned dish should do the trick. The effect is heightened if you combine nutmeg with foods high in tyramine such as mature cheese, pineapple, avocado, chocolate or cured meat. Tyramine stimulates the release of the very monoamines that nutmeg keeps active, resulting in a double dose of fun. Gastronomically and chemically everything comes together in the supper classic of macaroni cheese spruced up with posh cheese, smoked ham and spinach. Nutmeg is equally adept in sweet dishes. A rum, ginger and pumpkin cake with nutmeg frosting should hit the spot – pumpkin pie crossed with carrot cake on honeymoon in Barbados.

....

Florentine Macaroni Cheese

Nutmeg : 1
Milk : 150 ml
Bay leaf : 1
Parsley : a few stalks
Onion : a few slices
Peppercorns : 3
Butter : 2 tbsp
Plain flour : 1 tbsp
Comté cheese : 60 g
Parmesan : 60 g
Taleggio cheese : 60 g
Smoked cooked ham : 4 thick slices
Baby spinach : 150 g
White bread : 1 slice
Mustard powder : a large pinch
Dry macaroni . 250 g
Garlic : 1 clove
Mascarpone : 100 g
Parma ham : 2 slices
Salt and pepper : to taste

Preheat the oven to 200°C.

First off prepare your béchamel. Grate half the nutmeg into the milk, add a bay leaf, a few parsley stalks, a couple of slices of onion and a few peppercorns. Gradually bring to the boil, then take off the heat and when cool, strain out the solids.

Melt 1 tablespoonful of butter in a small pan. As soon as it has melted remove from the heat and stir in the plain flour. Gradually beat the infused milk into the roux paste. Return to the heat and bring to the boil, stirring all the while. Allow to boil for a few minutes to cook out the starch and your work is done.

Grate the Comté and Parmesan cheese and cut the Taleggio into small cubes.

Slice the smoked ham into 1 cm strips and roughly chop the baby spinach.

Cut the crusts from the slice of white bread and whizz up in a food processor to make some breadcrumbs. Mix these with half the Parmesan and half the Comté. Grate a little nutmeg into the breadcrumbs, season with pepper and add the mustard powder. Mix together.

Bring a large pan of water to the boil. Cook the pasta for a minute or so less than required. Drain and rinse with boiling water.

Rub a baking dish first with garlic and then with butter.

Add the remaining knob of butter to the large pan. Heat and when the butter is foaming, add the sliced ham. Cook for a minute over a medium heat then throw in the pasta with the remaining Comté and Parmesan cheese, together with the mascarpone and chopped Taleggio, and the béchamel sauce.

The cheese will slowly melt on to the pasta and ham. Stir and shake the pasta in the pan to ensure it is melting evenly. If the sauce is looking dry add some more milk.

When the cheese has melted, add the chopped spinach and stir into the pasta.

Pour the pasta into the serving dish. Cover with the sheets of Parma ham and sprinkle with the Parmesan breadcrumbs.

Cook in the oven for 10 minutes, finishing under the grill if necessary to brown the crust. Serve with a large glass of red wine.

Pumpkin Cake with Nutmeg Frosting

Clove : 2
Cinnamon : ½ stick
Nutmeg : ½
Ginger root : 4 cm
Butter : 100 g
Eggs : 2 eggs, beaten
Brown muscovado sugar : 150 g
Self-raising flour : 150 g
Baking powder : 1 tsp
Salt : a large pinch
Walnut pieces : 75 g
Sultanas : 75 g
Dark rum : 75 ml + a tablespoon
Pumpkin (or butternut squash) : 250 g
(peeled and grated weight)

FROSTING
Icing sugar : 100 g
Cream cheese : 200 g
Butter : 85 g
Vanilla extract : ½ tsp
Nutmeg : ¼

Preheat your oven to 180°C. Butter a small roasting dish and line with baking paper.
In a pestle and mortar or spice grinder turn the cloves and

cinnamon into powder. Grate the nutmeg and finely chop the ginger.

In a food processor, beat the butter until fluffy. Add the sugar and beat together. While the motor is running gradually pour in the beaten egg.

Sift together the flour, spices, baking powder and salt. Add to the egg mix then fold in the walnut, chopped ginger, sultanas and rum. Finally stir in the grated pumpkin or butternut squash.

Pour the cake mix into a tin and bake for 40 minutes or until the top is springy.

Allow the cake to cool for 5 minutes, then turn out on to a rack. Spike the cake with a skewer and sprinkle with some more rum while warm. Leave to cool.

Meanwhile make the frosting by beating together the icing sugar, cream cheese and butter. Add the vanilla extract and grated nutmeg and beat in.

Slather the cake with frosting. Serve small pieces dusted with a little more nutmeg as after-dinner petit fours or big pieces for afternoon tea in bed.

....

PEPPER

The ubiquitous peppercorn is the undisputed champion of the spice world. A few turns of the pepper mill will lift almost any dish. The power of pepper, however, is not restricted to purely culinary matters. It also enjoys a mighty aphrodisiac reputation – according to legend nothing heralds a good grinding more than a hefty pinch of pepper.

To secure a lady's ecstatic affection, the fabled Kama Sutra advises its readers to baste their privates in pepper and honey. *The Perfumed Garden* is equally enthusiastic on the subject. The Arab advisory commends an even more delicate placement of pepper, 'upon the head of your member', promising 'matchless enjoyment' for all involved. Those who fret about the size of said member can also benefit. The classic text prescribes pepper, honey, lavender, galangal, musk and ginger. Massage this paste into the nether regions, and watch with wonder as the skinny runt becomes 'large and brawny', capable of filling a lady with 'a marvellous feeling of voluptuousness'. Not to be sneezed at.

Aphrodisiac or no, the peppercorn has a unique and exalted place in history. Indigenous to India, pepper was one of the first traded commodities. As far back as 1213 BC pepper was being brought to Egypt. Rameses the Great, the legendary Ozymandias, was mummified with peppercorn stuffed in his nostrils. By Roman times the pepper trade was immense, employing a fleet of 120 ships. In the Middle Ages a monopoly on pepper funded the splendours of the Italian Renaissance. This monopoly drove Portugal, Spain and England to set sail around the world seeking new routes to the spice, sowing the seeds of five centuries of European colonialism. Wider availability turned the original black gold into an everyday essential. By 1700 even the distinctly plebeian Peter Piper could afford to pick a peck of pickled pepper – much to everyone's tongue-tangling mirth.

A peck is an imperial dry measure equivalent in volume to approximately 9 litres. With this amount of pepper at his disposal Peter Piper could get up to an awful lot of mischief, as the scientific evidence very much supports pepper's aphrodisiac reputation. The compound piperine is responsible for pepper's heat and also its hot reputation. Piperine stokes up the body's metabolism and increases the production of serotonin and beta-endorphins. A faster metabolism will generally improve energy levels, which as one might imagine is no bad thing for the carnal-minded. The increased production of serotonin and beta-endorphins is more specifically pleasure related. Serotonin combines the double whammy of brightening the mood and delaying the arrival of that gloriously sticky male moment. Which in itself must surely improve the mood of the fairer sex.

Beta-endorphins are the body's natural opiates, eighty times stronger than morphine. They are released in moments of extremis. Designed to soothe acute pain, endorphins also influence the opposite end of the pleasure spectrum, being largely responsible for the proverbial post-coital bliss. Logically, more endorphins should equal more bliss – and this is indeed the case. As for rubbing pepper on one's Peter Piper, it sounds jolly painful but perversely there is probably something in it. Piperine would certainly stimulate blood flow to the profane extremities, which in turn should indeed produce a brawny yet nerve-tingling performance. As Jane Fonda might say, 'no pain no gain' – but then again, perhaps 'feel the burn' is more appropriate.

When it comes to the kitchen, ignore Fonda's Law; pain is off-limits and the burn is to be avoided. A thoroughly civilised gentle heat will suffice. Pepper's uses are endless but perhaps the most prominent are in the seasoning of eggs, cabbage, pasta and potatoes, for which it is indispensable. Pepper's main flavour compounds all evaporate in air. To ensure optimum spice, always use freshly ground pepper and store peppercorns in an airtight container.

A great way to highlight this versatile spice is pepper and salt squid. Serve with a sweet chilli and saki dipping sauce and hopefully more painful preparations won't be required.

....

Black Pepper Baby Squid

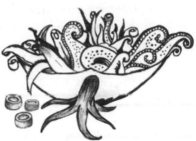

Baby squid : 250 g
Black pepper : 1 tbsp
Flaky sea salt : 1 tsp
Plain flour : 75 g
Cornflour : 75 g
Cayenne pepper : a pinch
Vegetable oil : for frying
Sake : 1 tbsp
Sweet chilli dipping sauce : 3 tbsp
Toasted black sesame seeds : 1 tsp
Finely sliced red chilli : 1 tbsp
Sliced spring onion : 1 tbsp

Wash the baby squid under cold running water, drain and pat dry. Remove the tentacles and ensure the squid is cartilage-free. Cut the squid into 1 cm-wide rings.

Pound the pepper and salt to a powder with a pestle and mortar. Mix with the flour, cornflour and cayenne pepper.

Heat clean vegetable oil in a pan until it is very hot. Then begin frying.

Dip the squid rings and tentacles in the black pepper flour, shake off excess and place in the hot oil.

Fry in small batches for about 4 minutes each, or until golden brown and crispy. Remove from the oil with a slotted spoon and place on kitchen paper to absorb the excess. Keep the cooked squid rings well spread out to ensure they remain crispy, and place in a warming oven while frying the rest.

Prepare the dipping sauce by simply mixing the sake with the sweet chilli sauce.

Serve the squid sprinkled with toasted black sesame seeds and the finely sliced red chilli and spring onion.

....

SAFFRON

The oldest aphrodisiac of them all, saffron has been on the job for well over 3,000 years. Spreading like a hot flush across the Mediterranean and Asia, the saffron crocus was at one point the most cultivated flower on the planet. Its bright red stigmas were worth more than gold, prized as religious offering, resplendent dye, traditional medicine, alluring cosmetic, gastronomic flourish and groin girder par excellence. Not bad for the sterile sex organ of a mutant flower.

Saffron's antiquity has burnished it with enough myth and mystery to fill an entire book. Minoan legend tells of unfortunate Jack-the-lad Krokus. Punching above his weight, he bagged a tricksy nymph called Smilax. Soon tiring of his besotted ways, Smilax gave our hero the heave-ho. Thoroughly unmanned, Krokus faded, wasting away until he was miraculously transformed into the first saffron crocus. Krokus's ardour is said to burn for ever in the flaming stigmas of this purple flower. Zeus, numero uno of the Greek gods, used saffron to abduct the beautiful princess Europa. Cunningly disguised as a white bull, he sneakily blew saffron up her nose. Suddenly besotted with this brazen bovine, Europa mounted her new best friend and was carried off to Crete for a spot of bestiality on the beach. I dare say she was thoroughly ashamed of herself the next morning.

I doubt Cleopatra was ever ashamed of her amorous extremes. This queen of the bedchamber would bathe in saffron-spiced water to sweeten long nights of Egyptian ecstasy. Probably the most expensive toilette in history: the finest saffron costs £10,000 per kilogram and she is said to have used half a cup of the stuff.

Saffron's mighty price tag seems more reasonable when you learn that over 150,000 hand-plucked flowers are required to produce each kilogram. Fortunately for the bon viveur on a budget only a pinch is required in most dishes. In food, saffron works in three ways, imparting the bittersweet scent and the flavour of fresh hay, and a resplendent golden colour. The active agent responsible for this riot of mellow yellow is a chemical compound called crocin. Crocin also appears quite capable of activating a slumbering libido. The exact mechanics remain mysterious but a team of inquisitive Iranian boffins has shown that male rats get their whiskers well and truly tickled by a dose of both saffron extract and crocin extract. Good news for all you love rats out there.

The culinary uses of saffron are multitudinous and rather varied. It is a central ingredient in some of the world's most celebrated savoury rice dishes: risotto Milanese, paella Valenciana and Hyderabadi biryani. It partners well with seafood, as in the incomparably fishy French bouillabaisse. But it is equally at home in desserts, partnered with poached pears or even rose water in Iranian ice cream. My ultimate saffron fancy is a fish pie that positively glows with aphrodisiac goodness: smoked haddock, asparagus and tiger prawns bound in a saffron sauce and topped with a nutmeg-spiced parsnip and potato mash. Serve with a casually dressed endive salad and a fat yellow Chardonnay.

Smoked Haddock and Saffron Fish Pie

Saffron : 15 strands
Milk : 500 ml
Bay leaf : 2
Cloves : 2
Smoked haddock loin : 300 g
Floury potatoes : 300 g
Parsnips : 200 g
Asparagus : 150 g
Cooked tiger prawns : 150 g (cooked and shelled weight)
Butter : 80 g
Plain flour : 2 tbsp
Nutmeg : ¼
Salt and pepper : to taste

Hydrate the saffron in 50 ml of hot water and leave to infuse for 5 minutes. Pour the milk into a pan add the bay leaves, cloves

and saffron water and heat until
the surface begins to shiver.

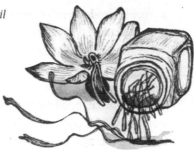

Cut the haddock into large
pieces, then place into the hot
milk. Remove the pan from
the heat and leave to cool.

Peel the potatoes, cut
into large chunks, then cook in
salted water until soft enough
to mash. Once cooked drain off the water and leave to mash
later.

Similarly, peel the parsnips, cut up and boil in water until soft.
Drain and reserve.

Blanch the asparagus in boiling water for 4 minutes, then
refresh under cold water. Chop into 3 cm lengths and set aside.
When the milk is lukewarm the fish should be lightly cooked.
Carefully remove the fish, discarding the skin, and place on the
buttered base of a small pie dish for two. Place the tiger prawns
and asparagus pieces over the fish. Strain the saffron milk and
reserve for use in the sauce and mash.

Prepare the saffron sauce by first melting half the butter in
a non-stick pan. When the butter begins to foam, add the plain
flour and beat together.

On a very low heat gradually beat in the saffron milk, adding
a little at a time to ensure that the sauce has an even consistency
at all times. Stop adding milk when the consistency is like single
cream, increase the heat a little and slowly bring the sauce to
the boil while stirring constantly. The sauce will thicken to the
consistency of thick double cream as it approaches boiling point.

Once it is boiling turn the heat up and let the sauce bubble for a few minutes to cook out the flour.

Beat in a little extra butter to give the sauce a rich sheen and season with salt and pepper. Pour the sauce over the fish and asparagus mix and stir gently to combine all the elements. The final process is to prepare the mash. Mash the potatoes by hand and blitz the parsnips in a food processor. Mix the parsnip purée into the potato and add the remaining butter. Season to taste with salt, pepper and lots of nutmeg and spoon over the pie filling.

The pie can be made in advance. When it is time to serve, simply plonk it in a hot oven (200°C) for 20 minutes to heat through and turn the topping a golden brown.

VANILLA

Vanilla is the kind of aphrodisiac you might want to marry. The floral scent and sweet flavour of vanilla are pure unadulterated fresh femininity. As an aphrodisiac it represents all that is good and wholesome and beautiful in love. Such things are hard won and highly prized; vanilla is a high-maintenance madam. Its production is expensive, difficult and very labour intensive. On a summer's day, dipping a perfectly ripe strawberry into a fluffy mound of vanilla Chantilly cream, I think it well worth the effort and cheap at the price.

What we know as vanilla is the pod and seeds from the tropical vanilla orchid. As with all orchids, the flower bears an uncanny resemblance to the tidy hoo-ha of a particularly well-groomed lady. Unlike most ladies, this flower opens for one day a year, is hermaphroditic, and with a helping hand is capable of self-fertilisation. The vanilla farmers must work fast, scuttling up ladders to hand-pollinate each flower before the end of the day. Once fertilised, the orchid produces a long seed pod which contains the precious seeds, or beans as they are more commonly known. Nine months later the pods are ready to harvest. The plucked pods are first blanched in hot water for a few minutes, then wrapped in wool and left to sweat in the sunshine for up to ten days. The flavours and aromas develop under these steamy conditions. The pods are then dried and conditioned for a further three months.

Indigenous to the jungles of southern Mexico, it was the Totonac people who first devised the laborious techniques of vanilla production. The only difference is that in the jungle Melipona bees and small humming birds pollinate the orchids. According to Totonac legend, the vanilla orchid is a divine aphrodisiac, an incarnation of Xanat, daughter of the fertility goddess. She fell in love with a handsome Totonac youth. As her divinity prevented her from marrying her human beau, she transformed herself into the vanilla orchid to provide pleasure and sensuality to her mortal love. The Totonacs used vanilla in xocolatl, an aphrodisiac hot drink made with cacao and chilli. The custom spread to the Mayans and Aztecs. The Spanish conquistadors wrote of the great Aztec king Montezuma's voracious thirst for this brew and boggled at his harem-hushing prowess. Sampling it themselves, the conquistadors were impressed enough to send it on the first ship back to Spain.

This exotic combination of vanilla and chocolate was a sensation in the old world. The aphrodisiac effect of hot chocolate was largely attributed to vanilla as opposed to chocolate. Medically it was regarded as 'warming', with correspondingly hot effects on the libido. Soon, doctors across Europe were prescribing vanilla to ensure male potency. In 1762 Bezaar Zimmerman, a German doctor, claimed that he had transformed 'no fewer than 342 impotent men, (who) by drinking vanilla decoctions, had changed into astonishing lovers of at least as many women'. The gourmet president Thomas Jefferson is credited with introducing vanilla to the USA. As before, vanilla was an absolute hit. In the American Dispensatory, readers were advised to use vanilla to 'stimulate the sexual propensities'.

Tried and tested over thousands of years, folk remedies are rarely without foundation. Vanilla is no exception. Vanilla increases levels of adrenaline, the chemical responsible for the racing heart, sweaty palms and increased blood pressure of intense attraction. It is mildly addictive, so may be responsible for vanilla's inexorable rise to its current position as the world's favourite flavouring. The aroma of vanilla is as much part of its gourmet allure as its flavour; it is also a key part of its saucy appeal. Dr Alan Hirsch, an expert in all matters nose and tongue, identified vanilla as the mature man's sexiest scent. A whiff of vanilla was found to be just the thing to get blood pumping to the nether regions. Millions of pounds of vanilla-tinged perfume sales confirm his findings.

The bon viveur trying to vajazzle with vanilla should stick to the real deal. Vanilla pods are expensive but offer so much more fragrant complexity than artificially produced vanilla extract. There are three main cultivars of vanilla: Mexican, Bourbon and Tahitian. Mexican vanilla, still grown by Totonac Indians, is generally regarded as the finest of the three. Its spicy tones are richer and more earthy than the fruity Tahitian and mellow Bourbon. A well-matured pod should be pliable with a deep oily-brown colour and a glittery sheen. The fragrance should be heavenly. The English were the first to use vanilla as a stand-alone flavour. Hugh Morgan, apothecary to Elizabeth I, is credited with this gastronomic innovation. The French grudgingly honour the great British custard with the title crème anglaise. As fantastic as custard can be, I find vanilla most fantastic in its purest form, whipped into cream and icing sugar to create the incomparable Chantilly cream. If you have to smear a lover with anything, this is what you want to be licking off. Like a pair of lacy French knickers on an English schoolboy, it sexily transforms the stiff-upper-lipped meringues and strawberries of Eton Mess. Serve with a sprinkle of strawberry dust and a glass of pink champagne. Resistance will be futile.

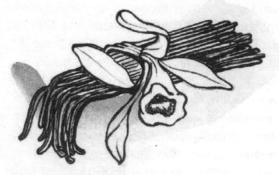

Eton Mess

Strawberries : 400 g of small strawberries
Eggs : 2
Caster sugar : 120 g
Tahitian vanilla : 1 pod
Whipping cream : 250 ml
Icing sugar : 1 tbsp or to taste

STRAWBERRY DUST

Remove the hulls from 200 g of the strawberries. Slice the strawberries finely and arrange flat on a baking tray lined with non-stick baking paper.

Place in the oven on its lowest setting, ideally around 75°C. Cook for 3 hours until completely dry.

Put the dry strawberries in the freezer for 15 minutes. Remove and grind to a powder in a coffee grinder or pestle and mortar. Store in an airtight container.

MERINGUES

Preheat the oven to 150°C.

Carefully separate the yolks from the egg whites.

Pour the whites into a very clean metal bowl and add a third of the caster sugar. Whisk vigorously until the whites have formed soft peaks.

While whisking gradually add another third of the sugar, 1 teaspoon at a time, whisking until the whites form stiff peaks.

Using a metal spoon fold in the remaining sugar, taking care not to knock out any air from the meringue mix.

Place 4 large dollops of meringue mix on to a baking tray lined with non-stick baking paper. Place in the oven and bake for 15 minutes.

Reduce the temperature to 110°C and cook for a further 2½ hours until very crisp and dry.

Place on a baking tray to cool.

CHANTILLY CREAM

Cut the vanilla pod lengthways and scrape out the sticky seeds with the back of a knife. I recommend using Tahitian vanilla. Its fruity qualities complement strawberries perfectly.

Stir the vanilla into the cream, and sweeten to taste with icing sugar.

Whip the cream until it forms soft peaks.

MAKING THE MESS

Hull and slice the remaining 200 g of strawberries.

Using a bread knife cut the meringues into 2 cm chunks.

Fold the meringue and strawberries into the whipped cream.

THE APHRODISIAC ENCYCLOPAEDIA

*Pile the mess into two champagne coupes and sprinkle
liberally with strawberry dust.*

Vanilla Panna Cotta with Poached Peach and Strawberries

Peach : 1
Strawberries : 6
Sweet Moscatel white wine : 175 ml
Honey : 1 tbsp
Vanilla pod : ½
Gelatine : 1½ leaves
Whole milk : 125 ml
Double cream : 125 ml
Caster sugar : 1 tbsp
Icing sugar : for dusting

*Remove the stone from a ripe peach and cut into halves. Remove
the hulls from the strawberries and cut into quarters.*

*Pour the wine, honey and split vanilla pod into a saucepan.
Heat gently until the honey has dissolved.*

*Put the peach halves in the syrup, cover and simmer gently
for about 15 minutes. Add the strawberries for the last 5 minutes.
The peach should be tender but not soft. If the peach halves are
not totally covered by syrup make sure you baste and turn the
fruit a few times while cooking.*

*Remove the peach halves, strawberries and vanilla from
the syrup, turn the heat up and reduce the liquid by half at a
fast rolling boil.*

Peel the skin from the peach halves. It should come

*away easily, having been loosened by the poaching
process.*

Soak the gelatine leaves in cold water to rehydrate.

*Pour the milk and cream into a small pan. Split the vanilla
pod, scrape out the seeds and put both pod and seeds into the
creamy milk.*

*Bring the creamy milk to a light simmer, then add sugar to
taste.*

*Squeeze any excess moisture from the hydrated gelatine, then
add to the creamy milk. Remove the pan from the heat, take out
the vanilla pod, and stir gently until the gelatine has dissolved.*

*Pour the panna cotta mix into two dariole moulds or
ramekins. Chill the panna cotta in the fridge for at least an hour
or until it has set.*

*To serve, turn out each panna cotta on to a shallow bowl.
Place the poached peach half alongside with a scattering of
poached strawberries. Spoon the cool syrup over both peach and
panna cotta. To finish, dust with a little icing sugar.*

WASABI

There is something rather magical about wasabi. The very best
grows on the sacred slopes of Mount Fuji in the shallows of constantly flowing mountain streams. A hefty lump of luminous
light green, the wasabi root's proportions are something even
the Incredible Hulk would be proud to find in his underpants.
Pulp wasabi using the traditional shark-skin grater and you have
culinary Semtex. The glowing green paste will blow you away.

It is blisteringly and bewilderingly hot. The pungency sears the nose with incapacitating fury, then evaporates as swiftly as it arrived. One can hardly believe there is no lasting damage. The palate is miraculously refreshed and cleansed, washed with wasabi's delicate, sophisticated flavour. There may be tears in your eyes and your nerves may be jangling, but the invigoration is palpable. The world seems brighter and more wonderfully alive than a moment ago. The Japanese are quite correct: how could wasabi not be an aphrodisiac?

Wasabi explodes across the senses in the same way as chilli. It smites the sensitive heat sensors with an almighty hit of isothiocyanate, the same active ingredient that gives mustard its bite. Unlike capsaicin in chilli, which is a clinging oil, wasabi's firepower is water-soluble and easily extinguished. The trauma passes speedily as saliva deactivates and disperses isothiocyanate almost immediately. Despite the brevity of the onslaught, alarm bells ring in the central nervous system. Endorphins are deployed to wash the body with pleasure. The heart rate jumps and blood vessels dilate as the body mobilises for evasive action. From evasive to invasive in a matter of moments, the bells are silenced and, ring-a-ding-ding, tingling senses are reinterpreted as sudden arousal. The pinnacle of sashimi presentation is nyotaimori, female body presentation. Slivers of raw fish are artfully arranged over the naked body of a well-scrubbed beauty. It is an exercise in self-restraint. Reining-in wasabi-induced urges requires every ounce of the impeccable self-control for which our oriental friends are rightly famous.

Wasabi has additional long-term Boy's-Own benefits. It is a member of the cruciferous family of vegetables that includes cabbage, broccoli, radish, horseradish and Brussels sprouts. All of these vegetables share a substance called indole-3-carbinol, which has a significant anti-oestrogenic effect. Specifically, it diminishes the amount of female hormones swilling around middle-aged men, boosting testosterone and bolstering libido. Load up on these veggies three times a week and the mature man can re-release the amorous hits of youth. Embarrassing for offspring, but great for mums and dads.

Horseradish is a close relative of wasabi and shares its aphrodisiac power. Much of the wasabi used in the West is in fact a mix of powdered horseradish, mustard and green food colouring. Although horseradish has similar heat it is no substitute for the authentic taste of real wasabi. When buying wasabi in a shop always check the label to make sure you are getting the genuine article. Fresh wasabi is uncommon outside Japan, so you will usually find it in powder or paste form. There is no advantage to either as the paste is just rehydrated powder. The classical sushi combination of wasabi and light soy sauce can be stretched to create a vibrant dressing for a salad of seared salmon with watercress and avocado. It combines well with honey to create a delicious punchy glaze for roast salmon or even gammon. My heart, however, is forever smitten with the fusion dish of wasabi-tinged tuna tartare. This can be served on cucumber slices as hors d'oeuvres or as a full-blown starter with a pile of chilled soba noodles. Don't scrimp on the quality of your raw tuna as this is essential to the success of the final dish.

....

Tuna Tartare with Soba Noodle Salad

Spring onion : 2
Raw tuna : 150 g (the very best quality)
Avocado : 1
Ginger root : ½ tsp (very finely grated)
Light soy sauce : 2 tbsp
Sesame oil : 1 tbsp
Wasabi paste : 1 tsp
Sushi vinegar : 1 tbsp
Furikake seasoning : 1 tsp

Finely slice the white part of the spring onions and finely chop the tuna and avocado. Mix with the all the remaining ingredients and set aside for the flavours to infuse. If you can't find furikake seasoning (which is a mix of black and toasted white sesame seeds with nori seaweed and red shiso leaf) just use toasted sesame seeds.

SOBA SALAD

Dry soba noodles : 100 g
Rocket : a good handful
Spring onion : 1
Carrot : 1
Cucumber : ¼
Radishes : 4
Light soy sauce : 3 tbsp
Mirin : 3 tbsp
Tabasco : ½ tsp

Cook the soba noodles as instructed until al dente, plunge into cold water and rinse twice to wash out all the remaining starch. Squeeze dry and place in a bowl. Finely slice the rocket and the spring onion. Slice the carrot and cucumber and radishes into fine strips and toss with the soba noodles. Mix the soy sauce with the mirin and Tabasco, then stir through the salad. To serve, place the noodle salad in two shallow bowls. Use an oiled chef's ring to clear a space in the middle of each salad and fill with tuna tartare. Remove the ring to reveal neat cylinders of tuna tartare. Serve with a crisp Alsace Riesling or warm sake.

Wasabi and Ginger Salad Dressing

Ginger : 2 tsp
Wasabi paste : 2 tsp
Light soy sauce : 3 tbsp
Honey : 2 tsp
Rice vinegar : 1 tbsp
Toasted sesame oil : 1 tbsp

Grate the ginger to form a paste, then whisk together with all the other ingredients. If you want a fibre-free dressing, allow the flavours to infuse for at least an hour, then sieve out the ginger. Serve with seared salmon or seared beef in a peppery salad.

Nuts, Seeds and Grain

ALMONDS

Almonds have long been regarded as both a symbol of love and a potent aphrodisiac, inciting men and exciting women in equal measure. Hirsute strongman Samson wooed dishy, deceitful Delilah with bouquets of flowering almond branches – not such a fine idea as it turned out. Swashbuckling French scribbler Alexandre Dumas swore by their fortifying properties, diligently putting away a bowl of almond soup before taking his squeeze, Mademoiselle Mars, to the moon and back.

Greek mythology tells of Phyllis, a beautiful Thracian princess. She met and fell in love with the warring Athenian prince Demophon, as he travelled home from Troy. They were to be married, when news of his father's death called Demophon back to Athens on the eve of their wedding. Demophon swore to return by the next full moon and fulfil his promise to marry Phyllis. Months passed without word. Distraught and bereft of hope, Phyllis hanged herself, whereupon the gods, moved by her sadness, turned her into the first almond tree. A disastrously delayed Demophon returned to find his beloved now a leafless, flowerless tree. Desperate with sorrow he embraced the tree, which spontaneously, and romantically, burst into flower. The ancient Greeks took this as a tale of great love and the almond tree has been prized as a symbol of romance in Greece ever since.

In the Middle East the almond is both widely cultivated and particularly revered. Commended by Arab sexologist Sheikh al-Nafzawi in his famed instructional tome *The Perfumed Garden*, they are duly dished out to perk things up at nuptials across Arabia. The Saudi government, impressed by the almond's claim to fame, has conducted the only systematic study into their use as an aphrodisiac. Researchers at King Saud University put mice on an almond-rich diet, and observed with wonder as their rodent sperm became impressively hyperactive. Backing up the mouse research is some heavyweight nutritional support, showing almonds to be a rich source of vitamin E. Vitamin E is essential to healthy sexual function. When deprived of this essential nutrient males experience serious nut shrinkage, whilst females are rendered infertile; fortunately both predicaments are easily alleviated by a healthy helping of vitamin E-rich almonds.

When it comes to preparing almonds, there is a wealth of ways to sneak them into one's nosh. As a key ingredient in baking, ground almonds feature widely in patisserie, perhaps most notably in the Italian amaretti cookies. In north India ground almonds are used extensively to thicken curries, such as the ubiquitous Korma. Whilst these are admirable uses for this estimable nut, I think it comes into its own at the very start and very end of a meal; smoked or devilled almonds make a sublime cocktail snack and in the form of marzipan-stuffed apricots and raspberry macaroons they make exquisitely perfect petits fours.

Devilled Almonds

Cayenne pepper : a pinch
Smoked paprika : a pinch
Black pepper : a pinch
Cumin : a pinch
Sea salt : 3 pinches
Honey : 1 tsp

Sunflower oil : 1 tsp
Blanched almonds : 200 g

*Make a smooth paste with the cayenne, paprika, black pepper,
ground cumin, sea salt, honey and a little sunflower oil.*

*Coat the blanched almonds in the spice paste and leave to
absorb the flavours for a couple of hours.*

*Dry-fry the almonds in a hot non-stick pan for 5–10 minutes,
agitating and stirring to make sure they do not burn.*

Remove from the heat and leave to cool.

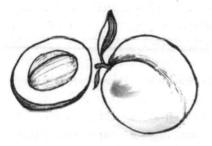

Marzipan-Stuffed Apricots

Blanched almonds : 100 g
Icing sugar : 100 g (and extra for dusting)
Amaretto liqueur : 1 tsp
Fresh apricots : 6
Flaked almonds : 1 tsp

*In a food processor, finely grind the blanched almonds, then add
the icing sugar and a teaspoon of amaretto liqueur. Continue*

to blend until the ingredients form a smooth paste – this is the marzipan.

Cut each apricot in half around the middle of the fruit. Remove the stone and the fill the pit of each half with the fresh marzipan.

Sprinkle the stuffed apricots with some toasted flaked almonds and dust with a little icing sugar.

Raspberry Macaroons
(makes about 10 macaroons)

Ground almonds : 150 g
Caster sugar : 150 g
Crème de framboise : ½ tsp
Egg whites : 2 medium-sized eggs
Whipping cream : 100 ml
Raspberries : 150 g
Icing sugar : for dusting

Preheat the oven to 200°C, and line a baking tray with non-stick baking parchment.

Place the ground almonds and sugar in a food processor, blitz to combine and whilst still running, gradually add the crème de framboise and the egg whites, adding only enough so that the mixture just holds together. Be careful not to overwork the almonds as their oil will begin to be released.

Shape the mixture into walnut-sized balls, place on the baking tray and flatten slightly.

Bake in the top of the preheated oven for 15 to 18 minutes. Once cooked, transfer the macaroons to a cooling rack.

*To serve the macaroons, slice them in half across the
width and fill with stiff whipped cream and a couple of fresh
raspberries. To finish, dust with a little icing sugar.*

....

CHOCOLATE

Chocolate is another much-hyped heavyweight of the aphrodisiac world. Its early history lies in the steamy forests of
Central America. The Mayan and Olmec civilisations got their
meso-American rocks off quaffing a frothy bitter drink called
xocolatl. This early drinking chocolate was made from the
roasted and then fermented beans of the god-food or cacao tree
with added chilli. The special properties of the cacao bean were
enjoyed across Central America. In Mayan wedding ceremonies
the happy couple would toss back a glassful to liven up the
night ahead. Aztec potentate Montezuma is said to have put
away fifty glasses a day to steel himself for sultry nights with
his extensive harem. He prized cacao above silver and gold, de-
manding it as tribute from his vassal states. Marauding Spanish
conquistadors were most perplexed when, on breaking into the
Aztec treasure chamber, they found not gold but cacao beans.
The beans were sent back to Spain with the rest of the booty and
so began the Western world's love affair with chocolate.

The Spanish sweetened the drink with sugar and quickly
agreed that chocolate was much easier to pronounce than
xocolatl. Chocolate fever swept across Spain like the clap and
within a few years was inspiring expensive nights of naughtiness across the whole of Europe. Venetian passion plunderer

Casanova declared it the 'elixir of love' whilst French ladies of ill repute perked up their drunken clients with restorative pots of chocolatey goodness. Bizarrely, it is the fun-phobic Quakers of un-merry England we have to thank for the world's first chocolate bar. In 1847 Fry & Sons of Bristol used the Van Houten method to split the ground chocolate bean paste into solids and butter. They then recombined them with sugar, and chocolate as we know it was born.

Today chocolate's saucy reputation is as entrenched as ever. Ladies seem particularly partial. My occasional furtive forays into the forbidden handbag have proven chocolate to be as essential to female happiness as lipstick, painkillers and strange cotton-wool objects which remain a mystery. Like most of the male world, every Valentine's Day I trot off to my favourite chocolatier and procure a box to woo my special lady.

A well-made truffle melting on the tongue is a deeply sensual experience not to be sniffed at. A nose around chocolate's nutritional properties reveals some rather inspirational findings. A team of British scientists recently discovered that chocolate raises pulses more effectively than a passionate kiss. Cocoa solids in chocolate contain three aphrodisiac suspects: theobromine, PEA (phenylethylamine) and tryptophan. Theobromine raises the heart rate and dilates the blood vessels in exactly the same way as sexual arousal. PEA occurs naturally in the brain in trace quanties that surge during orgasm and during the first flush of love. It is a bit opaque whether the PEA in chocolate can make the long trip from tummy to brain before metabolising. Dissolving chocolate on the tongue or snorting cocoa powder are probably the best ways to bring this love drug to the brain. Tryptophan breaks down into serotonin which, when it surges in the brain as it does during sex, creates a blissed-out sense of well-being.

With this much smoke there simply has to be some sort of sexual incendiary smouldering away in a bar of dark chocolate. Add the nutrition to the evidence in millions of female hand-bags and you have a mighty persuasive case.

The Aztecs and Mayans spiced their drinking chocolate with chilli and vanilla, two other equally aphrodisiac ingredients. Chocolate has a curious chemical romance with chilli, allowing you to take far more chilli than expected. Surprisingly delicious and as far from cocoa-at-bedtime as could be, this is pure sexual chocolate. Alternatively, dodge the Valentine's Day chocolate tax by preparing some sumptuous Chambéry chocolate truffles, guaranteed to melt your loved one's heart with extra points for effort.

Aphrodisiac Hot Chocolate

Whole milk : 600 ml
Vanilla pod : 1
Nutmeg : ¼
Red chilli : ½ mild chilli
Dark chocolate (minimum 70% cocoa solids) : 100 g
Sugar : to taste

Pour the milk into a pan.

Split the vanilla pod, scrape out the seeds and add to the milk.

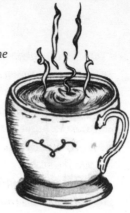

Grate the nutmeg into the milk and add the finely chopped chilli.

Heat gently, whisking the ingredients together so all the flavours infuse into the milk.

Shave the dark chocolate into wafer-thin slices using a vegetable peeler.

Stir the chocolate into the hot milk and allow to melt. Do not boil.

Strain out any solids and pour the hot chocolate into glasses. Serve immediately. Add sugar to taste.

Chambéry Truffles
(makes 20 truffles)

Vegetable oil : 1 tsp
Caster sugar : 100 g
Flaked almonds : 50 g
Lemon juice : a squeeze
Dark chocolate : 350 g
Double cream : 120 ml

Brush a metal baking tray with the vegetable oil.

In a heavy saucepan melt the caster sugar and heat until it reaches 130°C. Add the flaked almonds and squeeze of lemon juice and pour on to the greased baking tray.

Allow the praline to cool then break into pieces and grind to a powder in a food processor.

Chop the chocolate into small pieces. Add one third to a bowl, heat the cream to boiling point and add to the chocolate.

Let the cream and chocolate stand for a minute, then whisk
vigorously together. Add three quarters of the praline powder
and mix again.

Pour the truffle filling into a tray and chill in the fridge for an
hour.

Using a teaspoon, scoop out the filling and shape by hand
into 20 balls.

Place the truffles in the freezer for a further 2 hours to set.

Remove the truffles from the freezer and allow to warm for 10
minutes.

Gently heat the remaining chocolate in a bowl set over
simmering water.

Dip the truffles in the melted chocolate one by one, coating
them completely.

Carefully remove each truffle from the chocolate with a fork,
sprinkle with the remaining praline powder, and place on non-
stick baking parchment to set.

OATS

On a chilly Scots morning, nothing prepares for a Highland
fling like a steaming bowl of porridge. The oat groat is the
most humble and hearty of aphrodisiacs. Unlikely to wow with
exoticism or expense, oats thrive in cool damp climes and cost
next to nothing. It is rugged manly mystique and nutritional
nosebag that puts horse-feed on the bon viveur's aphrodisiac
high table.

Oats have long been associated with virility. Since the

Republic of Rome, the reckless rutting of young bucks has been fondly described as the sowing of wild oats. I have always taken the phrase to imply that a man has a certain amount of flighty seed that needs to be pumped out before he gets to the good dependable family-forming stuff. The sensible chap rattles through this froth in emotionally undemanding relation-ships with innkeeper's daughters, showgirls and the occasional bored housewife. Once the good stuff begins to flow, the sage stud moves on to marriage material. Not the most modern of views perhaps, but science is in full support of oats' manly association.

The extract from green oat straw has been shown to free up testosterone in both men and women, fuelling the desire for a roll in the hay. Once rolling, this extract is said to fight floppiness, and stops any half-cocked explosions from the old trouser cannon. Oats are pretty nutritious but the source of this goodness is rather more particular. Oats have a unique set of phytoalexins which act as a natural defence to deter rampant ruminants. These chemicals are known as avenanthramides and are present as much in oats as in green oat straw.

The Food and Drink Administration of America acknowledg-es that oatmeal is an effective anti-itching remedy. Rub it on a nettle sting and you will see the soothing avenanthramides in action. When eaten, oats act as a mild anti-histamine. As we saw with cheese, histamines speed lovers towards the delirium of orgasm. A mild dose of anti-histamines should keep this speed-ing within acceptable limits, steadying overexcitable libidos. Wise men say the journey is as important as the destination, and I say it is terribly rude to arrive at a party too early.

The same avenanthramides are responsible for oats' anti-impotence claims. A study at Tufts University in Boston has shown a direct correlation between avenanthramide levels and privates sector production of nitric oxide. Nitric oxide is absolutely fundamental to sex, providing the righteous rigidity of resplendent arousal. Released from artery walls on stimulation, nitric oxide causes blood vessels to dilate. The floodgates open and blood rushes in. The exit points, however, remain unaffected. The blood backs up, the pressure builds, and organs swell rudely with up to ten times as much blood as normal. Invest in a bowlful of porridge and hydraulic perfection is yours.

Although cheap, oats can be unexpectedly delicious. For gastronomic inspiration, look to the lochs and glens of bonny Scotland. Oats are as much part of Scotland's culinary heritage as whisky and haggis. I have happy memories of triumphantly landed trout tossed in oatmeal and fried in butter on a Hebridean Aga. Similarly, oatcakes are the perfect austere foil for a luxurious slice of smoked salmon. At breakfast, oats should be your cereal of choice. They are hot stuff in a bowl of steaming porridge with bananas, brown sugar and single cream. In summer, switch to the toasted oat super-muesli of granola. Mix with a wee dram, a drizzle of heather honey, some raspberries and a dollop of cream to create cranachan (often incorrectly called athol brose) – the bon viveur's luxurious oaty answer to the dourness of watery porridge.

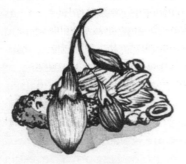

Oat and Goji Granola

Heather honey : 2 tbsp
Maple syrup : 50 ml
Sunflower oil : 1 tbsp
Rolled oats : 200 g
Salt : a good pinch :
Pumpkin seeds : 25 g
Pine nuts (preferably not Chinese) : 25 g
Sesame seeds : 2 tbsp
Flaked almonds : 50 g
Hazelnut pieces : 25 g
Dried goji berries : 50 g

Preheat the oven to 150°C. Mix the honey, maple syrup and oil in a large bowl. Separately mix the oats and salt together, then pour into the honey and maple mix. Mix together thoroughly so the oats are completely coated.

Spread the granola evenly on to a baking tray and bake for 15 minutes.

Remove the granola from the oven. Flip it with a metal spatula and stir in all the remaining ingredients except the berries. Return to the oven and bake for another 15 minutes.

Remove from the oven and scrape on to a tray to cool, at which point add the goji berries. Serve the granola with yoghurt or milk. Stored in an airtight container it will keep for up to a month.

Hazelnut Cranachan

Oatmeal : 50 g
Demerara sugar : 15 g
Heather honey : 4 tbsp
Hazelnut pieces : 2 tbsp
Highland malt whisky : 40 ml
Double cream : 225 ml
Hazelnut oil : 2 tbsp
Raspberries : 125 g

Preheat the oven to 180°C. Mix the oatmeal with the brown demerara sugar, a tablespoon of honey and the hazelnut pieces. Bake for 8 minutes, stirring to ensure that the oats toast evenly. Turn the oats out to cool.

Warm the Highland malt whisky with the remaining honey, stirring until the honey dissolves.

Whip the double cream until stiff and stir in the hazelnut oil and honey whisky.

Roughly mash half the raspberries and pass through a sieve to remove the pips.

Fold the raspberry sauce, whole raspberries and toasted oats

into the cream. Serve in a champagne coupe with a sprinkling of
reserved toasted oats.

....

PINE NUTS

Pine nuts are the edible seeds hidden in pine cones. An ancient food source, pine nuts have been gathered since prehistoric times and are a cracking aphrodisiac. There are separate, distinct and enthusiastic traditions of pine nuttery in European, Asian and Native American culture.

Harvesting pine nuts is a bit of a bore. The pine cones are gathered in the autumn, left to dry, then whacked until they surrender their seeds. The seeds have a hard outer shell. This is removed by hand to reveal the pine nut we all know and love. European pine nuts come from the stone pine. They are thinner, longer and stronger flavoured than the plump Chinese pine nut, which comes from the Korean pine. In America, the domestic piñon is very much larger and typically sold in its shell as a snack food.

The history of the use of pine nuts as an aphrodisiac is extensive. The effects were well known to both the Greeks and Romans. In the highly informative *Loving Arts*, Pliny includes them in his list of titillating titbits. The second-century medical pioneer Galen recommends an aphrodisiac tonic of honey mixed with twenty almonds and a hundred pine nuts. Three consecutive nights of treatment and all sexual woes could be forgotten. The obvious success of this prescription led to its re-recommendation in *The Perfumed Garden* in the fifteenth century. In the same period a very similar recipe was making merry in Old England. Pokerounce was an aphrodisiac Christmas treat of toasted white bread spread with spiced honey and sprinkled with pine nuts. The British Museum's Harleian Manuscripts contain the following olde English recipe:

Take Hony, and caste it in a potte tyl it wexe chargeaunt y-now; take & skeme it clene. Take Gyngere, Canel, & Galyngale, & caste þer-to; take whyte Brede, & kytte to trenchours, & toste ham; take þin paste whyle it is hot, & sprede it vppe-on þin trenchourys with a spone, & plante it with Pynes, & serue forth.

In the Himalayan uplands of northern India, the chilgoza pine nut is gathered for 'medicinal' purposes. It is used across the subcontinent to stiffen wilting libidos and increase male potency. Not great ones for written history, Native Americans have kept their traditions more mysterious. The basin tribes of Utah and Nevada gathered pine nuts from sacred groves of trees. The harvest fed winter love, warming up wigwams on long chilly nights.

Pine nuts are nutritionally rich. They are a good dietary source of niacin, zinc and arginine, all of which are required for an active and satisfactory sex life. These properties are all very well but not particularly remarkable. The pine nut's stand-out nutritional feature is its rare ability to suppress the appetite. In Siberia, when food is scarce over winter, hunger is appeased with a handful of pine nuts or a spoonful of pine nut oil. Modern research has identified pinolenic acid as the active ingredient.

Pinolenic acid triggers the release of two appetite suppressants. The signals are beamed to the brain by the mysterious vagus nerve. Separate from the spinal column, the vagus nerve is a sensory superhighway running from the genitals to the brain via the stomach, nipples, throat and chest. Pinolenic acid trips the vagus nerve's gut switch. A message is sent to the brain to release oxytocin, dopamine and opioids, the chemical cocktail of the fat and happy.

Oxytocin contracts the stomach walls to create that full-belly feeling. It is also closely linked to sexual arousal and orgasm. Often called the 'love hormone', oxytocin not only produces the loss of appetite of intense attraction but also post-coital fluffy feelings, thoughts of marriage and happily-ever-after. Oxytocin is released in greatest volume at orgasm. After an hour or so levels drop, the stomach walls relax, and you are soon being mauled by the post-sex munchies. Dopamine and natural opioids are equally involved in the neurochemistry of love. Dopamine creates feelings of desire whilst opioids wash the brain with pleasure. All in all it is a powerful combination at the pine nut's command.

Whilst the vagus nerve is not fully understood by modern science, it is clearly used to transfer sexual responses. A study at Rutgers University demonstrated that women with spinal cord injuries and no feeling from the waist down were still responsive to genital stimulation and able to have orgasms. Physical stimulation was being signalled to the brain by the vagus nerve. The funny feeling in your stomach, erect nipples and light-headed rush of sudden sexual attraction are all the handiwork of the vagus nerve. When the nerve fires, all points along it are stimulated. Strangulation and orgasm cause the most intense response. The two can blur together with grisly results. In hanging, the over-stimulation of the vagus nerve is responsible for the jutting gibbet girder of angel lust. Similarly, sexual self-strangulation is simply the sybarite's quest for the ultimate vagus-enhanced orgasm.

On a first date a nice pesto is rather more acceptable than an S and M collar. Pine nuts are the kingpin of what must be the world's most aphrodisiac sauce. Garlic, Parmesan, pepper, basil and pine nuts are all aphrodisiac stars in their own right. This versatile Italian paste is equally at home in a sandwich, on simple pasta dishes, or mixed with breadcrumbs as a crust for lamb chops. If you are out to impress, serve up a savoury basil and pine nut cheesecake: essentially deconstructed pesto. The creamy filling is infused with fresh basil and crowned with toasted pine nuts, the base crushed oatcakes and Parmesan. Serve suavely with a fresh tomato salad and suppress the smug grin of the satisfied chef.

....

Pesto Genovese

Butter : 10g

Toasted pine nuts : 25g

Sweet basil : 25g (weighed with stems)

Grated Parmesan : 25g

Pine nut oil (or light tasting olive oil) : 75ml

Garlic : one small clove, crushed

Salt : a large pinch

Chilli flakes : a pinch (optional)

Pepper : to taste
Lemon juice : a squeeze (optional)

The choice of sweet basil is moot; if you have a magnificent bush of purple basil go ahead and give it a trim. Having said that, sweet basil has the highest levels of basil oil and so makes a particularly aromatic pesto. Similarly, pine nut oil will add to your pesto's aphrodisiac effect but can be easily substituted by a mild olive oil or almond oil. Garlic, chilli, lemon and pepper are all a matter of personal preference and taste – they should be added as you like.

Melt the knob of butter in a frying pan and over a low heat toast the pine nuts. Stir and shake the pine nuts frequently so they brown evenly. Once they are golden brown remove from the heat – this process should take about 5 minutes.

In a pestle and mortar or food processor crush the toasted pine nuts. Once mashed into an oily pulp add the basil leaves and grind into the nut purée.

When the basil has submitted, add the Parmesan and pine nut (or olive oil) and mash/blend into the pine nut basil paste.

Add the crushed garlic, salt, chilli flakes and pepper to taste.

If you are preparing your pesto for the fridge, squeeze in some lemon juice to help preserve the vibrant flavours and colours.

Pine Nut and Basil Cheesecake

Oatcakes : 75 g
Parmesan : 40 g
Black pepper : a good grinding
Butter : 30 g
Garlic : 1 fat clove, crushed
Ricotta cheese : 200 g
Mascarpone : 200 g
Eggs : 2
Sweet basil : a packed-down mug full of leaves
Olive oil : 1 tbsp
Pine nuts : 100 g

Preheat the oven to 170°C.

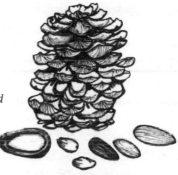

Crumble the oatcakes and grate the Parmesan, then mix together and season with lots of freshly milled pepper.

Heat the butter in a saucepan. Add the crushed garlic to the melted butter and sauté for a minute. Stir the garlic butter into the oatcake and Parmesan mix.

Press the oatcake mix into the bases of two wide biscuit rings (7 cm) or one small cake tin. The base should ideally be about ½ cm thick.

Beat together the ricotta and mascarpone cheese. Add the eggs one at a time and beat together vigorously.

In a pestle and mortar (or food processor) pound the basil leaves with a mild olive oil to make a thick smooth basil paste.

Add 3 tablespoons of paste to the cheese mix. Stir together and season with salt and pepper as required.

Pour the filling on to the oatcake bases and place in a pre-heated oven to bake for 40 minutes.

Meanwhile toast the pine nuts as described in the previous recipe.

When the cheesecakes are cooked remove them from the oven. Whilst still hot pour the pine nuts over the top, lightly pressing them into the top of the cheesecakes.

Allow the cheesecakes to cool completely and serve as a starter or summer lunch.

Anaphrodisiacs

The amour-intent bon viveur should be aware that some ingredients could be their undoing. Anaphrodisiacs are foods that stop lust in its libidinous tracks. These dietary cold showers helped celibate monks resist the devil's relieving hand and the weakness of the flesh. Worried that soldiers might make love rather than war, the powers that be, it is rumoured, spiked First World War army rations with anaphrodisiacs. Trench war and holy abstinence are not the natural millieux of the bon viveur, and anaphrodisiacs are to be avoided like the plague that they are.

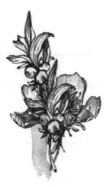

CHASTEBERRY

It is fortunate but not surprising that the chasteberry, *Vitex agnus-castus*, is not a popular spice. Well named, this plant's pant-calming effects have been known for an eternity. The Roman philosopher Pliny writes in his *Historia Naturalis* of *Vitex*'s ability 'to cool the heat of lust'. Athenian women during the chaste festival of Thesmophoria left their husbands' beds.

They resisted the lustful urges to return by sleeping on beds stuffed with *Vitex* leaves and twigs. Monks ground the berries on their food to ward off temptation, giving rise to its alternative name, monk's pepper.

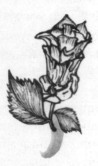

HOPS

Our next party pooper is of much more concern, being a key ingredient in what is, after water and tea, the world's most popular drink. Hops are an integral flavouring in almost all beer. The marketing men of big brewing have quietly covered up the fact that hops can torpedo your libido. The infamous brewer's droop is caused not by beer's modest alcohol content but by the unmanning properties of hops. They play havoc with your hormones, containing the most potent of phytoestrogens. I have often noticed that the inveterate ale guzzler sports not just the proverbial beer belly, but a handsome pair of teats too. The female hormones in hops may just be responsible. They are certainly strong enough to mess severely with a woman's reproductive system. After a few weeks in the fields, female hop-pickers experience acute menstrual problems and missed periods. As if all this wasn't bad enough, hops also send you to sleep. Following the sleepy work habits of hop cultivators, the folk remedy for insomnia is sleeping on a hop-filled pillow. No wonder women dislike pubs so much: who needs a big-breasted beer lump snoring away Saturday sex night? If you want post-pub passion make sure you inebriate yourself with wine or spirits – anything other than ale.

SOY

Soy is another anaphrodisiac no-no, confirming my meat-eater's antipathy to tofu and closet suspicions about limp vegan libidos. Soy is decidedly dampening to love's furnace and again the effects are mainly directed towards men. As with hops, powerful phytoestrogens are responsible, strangling a man's snake with the squeeze of an anaconda. In soy the phyto-estrogens are isoflavones and men should give them a wide berth if they value their testosterone. Contrary to popular opinion soy is not that widely eaten in the Orient. The group who eat the most soy are Japanese monks and they do so specifically to tame the distraction of sexual desire. Tofu, soya milk and edamame are all off-limits for lovers. The soya protein in limp lifeless vegan sausages is the white flag of sexual surrender. If you need to replace meat and milk, stick to pulses and oat milk. I am pleased to say that soy sauce escapes the embargo; the fermentation process knocks out the guilty isoflavones.

LETTUCE

Lettuce is an anaphrodisiac that acts on both women and men equally. It is a sedative, sending you off to the land of nod in next to no time – perfect for an after-lunch snooze on a hot summer's day, not so good for a postprandial poking. In Beatrix Potter's *Tale of the Flopsy Bunnies*, the little rabbits almost become Mrs McGregor's rabbit pie having fallen asleep following a slap-up lettuce lunch. Miss Potter's tales are not known for their scientific acumen but in this instance she is bang on the money. The milky sap released from the stalk of cut lettuce contains lactucarium, a sedative and analgesic similar to opium.

In ancient Greece, at the end of a splendid meal guests were often served lettuce soup. The idea was to send them blissfully off to the land of nod. The Roman emperor Domitian displayed his dark side by breaking with tradition and serving lettuce at the start of lengthy state banquets. It was forbidden to fall asleep in the emperor's presence, a crime that was punishable by death. Domitian was amused to see his drowsy guests struggle their way through dinner, knowing that nodding off would be fatal. To avoid a salad daze, stick to peppery leaves like rocket, mizuna and watercress, or bitter leaves like chicory and radicchio. Sprinkle with toasted pine nuts, dress with a garlic, honey and mustard vinaigrette and the great salad escape is complete.

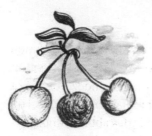

CHERRY

Cherries are a surprising anaphrodisiac. I have always thought they look rather sexy and the pout as you eject each cherry stone is undeniably suggestive. Also the phrase 'pop her cherry' has more than a hint of promise about it. For women, however, the smell of cherries is something of a turn-off. The studies by Alan Hirsch at the Chicago Institute of Smell and Taste recently revealed that the aroma of cherries decreased blood flow to the vagina by 18 per cent, the highest of all smells they tested. It does at least explain why Cherry Cola failed to catch on.